The Compleat Spanker

The Compleat Spanker
by Lady Green

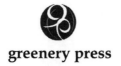

greenery press

Published in the United States by Greenery Press, 1447 Park Ave., Emeryville, CA 94608, www.greenerypress.com

ISBN 0-890159-00-X

Contents

Thanks to the citizens of Assville – the terrific folks who populate Usenet's soc.sexuality.spanking newsgroup – for their insights, encouragement, and willingness to share.

Thanks to all the loving, unforgettable people who have spanked me or been spanked by me through the years – Frank, Bob, Cheryl, Mic, Jaymes, Attila, Derek, Maryann, Daddy Drew and many more – and especially Tom, Barbara and Dossie.

Thanks to those who live and work around Greenery Press.

Special thanks to Snow White for providing a quiet place, away from Doc, Sleepy, Bashful and the gang, in which to finish this book.

And more thanks and love than I can possibly express to Jay, who loves (and spanks) me no matter how weird I get, and who makes my wonderful life possible.

1 Spanking and Me

O ne of my earliest memories is of sitting at the circus with my parents – I must have been four or so – and wondering what it would feel like to be spanked by the strong man.

As you can tell, my spanking fantasies go back a *long* way. I can hardly remember having any sexual fantasies at all that didn't include some form of spanking. And even now, although my interests have expanded to take in many other forms of consensual erotic pain play, spanking remains my first love.

Yet it took me a very long time to come to terms with this interest. Like many women, I found it easy to deny to myself that the fascinating thoughts and images that crowded my mind were sexual in nature. (Women, unlike men, cannot look down to gauge a phallic "barometer" of sexual arousal.) Thus, I was approaching thirty by the time I recognized that my spanking thoughts were actually sex fantasies.

Some of us are just a little slow, I guess.

And it took me even longer to recognize that lots of other people shared my interest. At the time, I was living a relatively conservative life in a small West Coast city, with very little exposure to erotic literature or photographs, and no access to the resources available in larger cities. And since my fantasies, like many other folks', were about nonconsensual spanking, I didn't realize that there were ways to act them out within the context of friendly and consensual sex play.

But eventually, the truth began to seep in: I was one of thousands, maybe tens or even hundreds of thousands, of people who had erotic connections with the act of spanking or being spanked. Suddenly, I began to see that I was virtually surrounded by spanking fans.

That was well over a decade ago. I began looking for and finding people to spank – and, later, people to spank me. I have spanked and been spanked by hundreds of people – men and women and transsexual, gay and straight and bi. I've used hands and paddles and hairbrushes and canes and birches and floggers and straps, and had them used on me. I've participated in light spankings that barely pinkened the skin, and heavy ones that left the backside bruised for weeks. And I think I can safely say that I've enjoyed every single one of them.

How this book came about

I've written several other books (under this name, and as "Catherine A. Liszt") that are more generally about erotic pain and power exchange play. My company, Greenery Press, has published several more. But I've come to realize that there's nothing out there, as far as I know, that offers detailed, specific information about spanking and spanking only. Spanking is certainly a precise enough craft, with exciting enough rewards, and with enough risk of physical and emotional damage, to merit a small book of its own.

Furthermore, I recognize that many people who enjoy erotic spanking don't consider themselves to be "into S/M," and thus may never look at the many excellent books on that topic. So this volume will, I hope, provide them with the information they need to practice safe and erotic spanking play.

My biases

I won't pretend to be completely open-minded about anything that involves smacking an ass. My biggest prejudice, of course, is against nonconsensual spanking. If you are reading this book looking for support for your practice of spanking a partner against his or her will in order to enforce "proper" behavior, you're out of luck; I believe nonconsensual spanking to be abusive behavior. If you are spanking someone against their will, or being spanked against your will, contact your local hotline for battering or battered partners immediately. (Contact information is listed in the Resource Guide at the back of this book.)

I also admit to looking with a very wary eye at the practice of spanking a partner as punishment for "mistakes" made in the real world, or out of a sense of anger or revenge. While I think that these practices *can* be done consensually and without harm, I think they are far riskier to the emotional well-being of the people involved and to the relationship between them than most folks realize. My suggestion is that unless you are in a very healthy relationship, and are a very skilled communicator with excellent personal boundaries, it's best to keep your spanking play within the realm of role-play and fun. Thus, I will not discuss in this book the idea of integrating spanking into the "real-world" part of your relationship.

I fantasize about this a lot, but I've found that for me and many folks, it's safer to keep in fantasy.

Lastly, I hope it goes without saying that spanking, like a fine brandy, is too rich and intoxicating a treat for children. I do not believe in spanking children, either as traditional punishment, or, of course, erotically. Please keep your adult spanking play between adults: do not spank, or be spanked by, anyone who is not of the age of consent in your state.

Don't worry – there's still *plenty* of hot, realistic spanking fun to be had between consenting adults who follow these guidelines! With love, creativity, skill and a few carefully selected toys, you have a lifetime of amazing sensations and astonishing emotional experiences ahead of you.

2 Who Spanks?

A *lot* of people are erotically attuned to spanking. So much so, in fact, that snickering references to erotic spanking have become a mainstay of television (I've counted spanking jokes on "Night Court," "Taxi," "The Nanny," "Third Rock from the Sun," "Frasier" and several others, and I don't watch much TV!). In less self-conscious times, spanking offered harmless titillation to generations of moviegoers (John Wayne's "McClintock!" is notorious) and readers (more than a few pre-Code comic books featured a comely moll getting walloped by a stern superhero). I'm also told that the less inhibited brand of romance novel often features threatened or real spankings of the heroine – I wonder how many women have been awakened to their own spanking interests by such "literature"? And of course, Madonna brought spanking firmly into the mainstream with her hit song "Hanky Panky."

I'm not a romance novel fan myself, but some readers' suggestions are listed in the Resource Guide.

So, when I hear someone ask the question "Is erotic spanking normal?" I'm a bit torn. If these people are asking "Is an interest in erotic spanking a statistical norm?" the answer is probably "No, but it's not highly unusual either." If, as is more likely, they're asking "But isn't it necessarily sick to want to give or receive pain?" I have an easier answer: "No, it isn't."

The experience of "pleasant pain" is familiar to many, perhaps most, people. (Not you? Think again: ever enjoyed the pleasant muscle ache of a good day's exercise, or the challenging burn of a spicy curry?) Many more, although they may not be consciously aware of it, also have some experience with erotically arousing pain:

biting, scratching, pinching, mild hair-pulling and hickeys have an honored place in many folks' sexual repertoire. If seeking out and/or eroticizing pain is "sick," then it's a "sickness" about as rare as the common cold.

Many of the "isn't it sick?" group seem to be particularly upset by the power imbalance implicit in spanking. After all, spanking is most often (rightly or wrongly) something done by a parent to a child, as a means of controlling the child's behavior and reinforcing the parent's authority over the child.

This is a trickier concern to answer. It's worth remembering, however, that many people enjoy erotic role-playing of various kinds, and that many of those games (coach and athlete, pirate and captive, teacher and student, owner and slave, "rapist" and "victim") include a pretended disparity in power. This enjoyment in no way means that the power disparity must extend into the day-to-day reality of the relationship. Nor is it true that a relationship with a well-bounded and consensual disparity of power is necessarily unhealthy, as long as both partners' needs for satisfaction and personal growth are being met.

So, in case you hadn't figured it out by now, I don't believe that the desire to spank or be spanked is by definition "sick." I do think it's possible for those desires to become so overwhelming or obsessive that they can constitute a sickness. Certainly, if your spanking interest:

Ask yourself: is the problem caused by external social messages against your spanking interest, or by your own guilt or self-hatred?

✋ Is interfering with your ability to do your work or maintain healthy relationships with your romantic partner, friends and/or family

✋ Is being expressed in a nonconsensual, bullying or abusive manner, or causing you to risk abuse or assault

✋ Is leading you to feel deeply guilty, ashamed, isolated or afraid

✦ Is causing you to spend more money than you can afford, or obsessing you to the point where you have trouble thinking about anything else

... then it may be time to get help in making spanking a more realistic and enjoyable part of your life. Check the Resource Guide in the back of this book for ideas about how and where to find such help.

Is spanking sex?

The answer to that question depends largely on the desires of the partners involved.

I feel fairly safe in saying that for most of you reading this, yes, spanking is sexual in nature. A few of the luckiest of you may be able to reach orgasm from spanking alone. Many others will use spanking as foreplay to more traditional sexual play such as intercourse or oral sex.

Yet there is a small subset of spanking fans out there who have no conscious erotic connection to the act of spanking or being spanked at all. They may simply be "sensation junkies," interested in testing their own abilities and exploring the outer edges of tolerable stimuli. Or they may use spanking as part of a lifestyle in which one person consensually gives another the right to control his or her behavior, using spanking as a form of discipline when the controlled partner goes astray.

Is spanking S/M?

This is a hotly controversial question among spanking circles. I've debated it on several occasions with spanking people, and what the discussion has almost always boiled down to is that their definition of "S/M" is very different than mine.

My working definition of S/M is "behavior in which the participants eroticize, or otherwise enjoy, sensations or emotions which would be unpleasant in a nonerotic context." (In this, I include the set of behaviors that are sometimes called "bondage & discipline" and "dominance and submission" – again, terms that are not universally defined even by their practitioners.) By this definition, I'd say that spanking is definitely S/M: getting smacked on the butt, in the absence of connection, intimacy and consent, is not a pleasant sensation for almost anyone... but a skillfully given, consensual, loving erotic spanking, even a very severe one, can be an extremely pleasant experience for those who like such things.

I've heard people state that their spanking interest is not S/M because "I don't enjoy the sensation of the spanking; I just like having my behavior controlled." Many people in the S/M community would say exactly the same. Enjoyment of pain is far from universal among S/M players; some accept the pain as a symbol of their devotion to their dominant, others accept it as a means of having their behavior controlled, and still others won't accept pain at all.

I've also heard spanking people reject the idea that what they do is SM because they are turned off by many of the outward symbols worn by some S/M people: the leather, the studs, the handcuffs, and so on. While these symbols are obvious means of publicly identifying oneself as "into S/M," they are far from universal. A great many S/M people, including me, seldom if ever wear or use such stuff (it's expensive and uncomfortable). If you were to attend a meeting of an S/M club, you would see a few people dressed in the traditional black leather uniform, a few more dressed as though they were on their way home from the office (because they are), and a few more dressed in jeans and sweatshirts, and a few more in costumes and drag, and quite a few miscellaneous types. Cutting yourself off from the resources of the S/M community because they dress funny is, I assure you, a mistake. (Important note: A significant number of the attendees

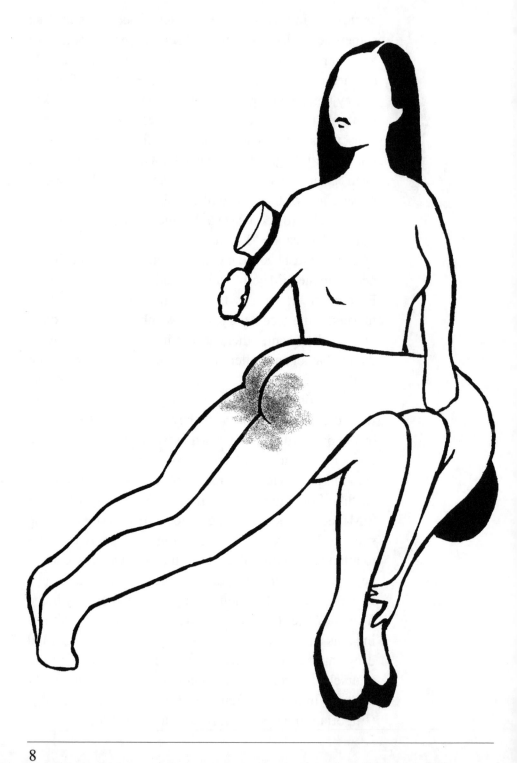

"Heavy" is jargon for physically or emotionally intense.

at the typical S/M club or party are interested primarily or exclusively in spanking.)

Finally, I think many spankers assume that S/M play is by definition "heavier" than spanking play. Not so. S/M play can be very light, teasing and erotic; spanking play can be very intense, painful and risky. (The reverse can, of course, also be true.) I suggest you define your interests by explaining what level of intensity you like, and not by relying on distinctions that may or may not exist.

Left: *a classic over-the-knee spanking, with a hairbrush.*

So, in my opinion and for the purposes of this book, yes, spanking is a subset of S/M play. You can take that as seriously or as scornfully as you like. A lot of the information you'll read here is gleaned from the collective experience of S/M players as well as spankers. While you may or may not ever desire to explore any form of erotic power exchange besides spanking, or to involve yourself in the S/M community as a whole, please do not close yourself off from many decades of experience, knowledge and possibilities.

3 Why Do We Like Spanking?

What's so great about getting whacked on the butt? For that matter, what's so great about whacking someone?

There are probably almost as many answers to these questions as there are spanking fans. Pain sluts, submissives, "babies," "brats," "puppies," and more enjoy getting spanked. Masters and mistresses, "coaches," "governesses," "mommies" and "daddies," shamans, and more enjoy doing the spanking. You probably share your particular motivations and fantasies with many other spankophiles, but your unique pattern of needs and desires and experiences is yours alone.

The physiology of spanking

Much of the motivation behind getting spanked is physiological: some aspects of spanking simply induce body responses which many people find pleasant. I don't think many people get into spanking in order to seek out these responses; instead, I think their fantasies, which I'll discuss later, lead them to try spanking, and they discover the physiological stuff as an added benefit. Some come to the point where they no longer need or want the context of the fantasy, but simply enjoy the physical sensations of the spanking, while others go on preferring to act out the emotional/role-playing aspects that surround the spanking play.

For a lot of folks, the physical sensations of spanking lead directly to arousal. As you'll see in the "Anatomy" chapter, there's a sound neurological reason for this. Certain parts of the butt share nerve groups, or dermatomes, with the genitals. Stimulation of these nerve groups "echoes" directly into the penis or clitoris, or more generally into the pubic area. Not everybody experiences this connection, but many people do; a few lucky ones can even reach orgasm solely from being spanked.

A second physiological goodie has to do, ironically, with the body's mechanisms for protecting you from intense sensation. When you receive a sound spanking, or any other intense physical or emotional stimulus, your brain releases chemicals called "endorphins" and "enkephalins." These naturally occurring substances are chemically similar to morphine. They reduce the pain and induce a state of mind which makes you feel drifty, giggly, serene, and/or just plain happy. Quite a few people engage in endorphin-seeking behavior: some ride roller coasters, some eat hot peppers, some run marathons, and some get their butts tanned. While I don't think too many people engage in spanking purely to get the endorphin rush, it's a very nice side benefit; some folks find it helps calm their minds and reduce their stress level for several days afterwards.

The psychology of spanking

Not that a few of us haven't tried it!

If all the rewards of spanking were physical, we'd simply smack our own butts. However, for most of us, spanking has at least as much to do with our emotions – with re-creating in the real world one of the deeply personal scripts that help make us who we are and that structure the way we relate to others. Often, these scripts describe someone who we're not allowed to be in the real world: the defiant brat, the acquiescent submissive, the dependent child... or, for tops, the strict parent, the cruel captor, the brusque owner. Within the protected boundaries of the spanking scene, we act out the roles that meet our most profound, most secret needs.

For many spankees, the "script" of spanking has to do with being controlled. They may or may not like the physical pain of being spanked, but they *do* like knowing that their spanker is administering the spanking as a symbol of her control.

Some control-oriented spankees identify as **brats**. Their style is defiant, insolent, resistant – they like the game that one of my friends calls "I'll pump it up, you take it down." Brat play often includes lots of little disobediences and impudences, which are designed to culminate in the top rolling up his sleeves and saying, in one way or another, "That's it, young lady, you've been asking for this."

A bottom is the person getting spanked – and, of course, also the part of them getting spanked.

Brat scenes can be a lot of fun, but they require particularly good boundaries and communication between the partners. It's a very bad idea to push a brat scene so far that the top genuinely loses her temper, or feels that she is being rejected or put down. It is particularly important in brat play for *both* top and bottom to have safewords, and to be willing to use them if anybody begins to feel that things have gotten too intense, anger-provoking, unsafe, or otherwise "real."

A safeword is a code word that someone uses to express that they really need things slowed down or stopped. See Ch. 5.

Other control-oriented spankees are **submissives**. For these folks, spanking is something they accept from their dominant because they know that giving a spanking pleases him. They are rarely resistant or mouthy; instead, they get their "script" from gamely doing their best to please.

If the cardinal weakness of brats is pushiness, a submissive's weakness can often be passivity. If you or your partner is submissive, be sure to check in often, outside the special world of the spanking scene, to be sure everyone's needs are getting met. A submissive may need a particularly large amount of reassurance that he is indeed pleasing his dominant – especially if he has had to safeword or otherwise express a limit.

Many spankees enjoy the ***catharsis*** of spanking. For a lot of folks, spanking offers an opportunity to release the pent-up angers, fears and frustrations which real life inevitably entails. While few people have the opportunity to rage, struggle, beg or cry in the outside world, the protected environment of a good spanking scene is a rare and magical place to let go of "stuffed" emotion, safe in the knowledge that our tops' strength will contain us, that we will harm nobody, and that we will still be loved after we release this difficult stuff.

Catharsis can be scary for all concerned: pity the poor top who thought he was just administering a nice simple straightforward spanking, and who suddenly finds himself having to contain and comfort a sobbing, incoherent wreck. If you suspect that you have a lot of pent-up emotion which is just waiting for a nice spanking in order to explode out of you, it's essential to warn your top first – to ensure that he gives his consent to be around such strong stuff, and that he's willing to support you as you release it.

Yet another category of spankee is the one who likes an ***ordeal***. For these people, taking a difficult spanking is a way of testing their own strength, courage and stamina. Afterwards, they report feeling strong, centered and powerful: they've taken what the world has to dish out, and it hasn't broken them. (I've heard this phenomenon referred to as "masochismo.")

A term coined by my friend Sadie Damascus.

Ordeal-seekers can be a bit of a trial for a top. Aside from the issue of wearing out your arm and breaking your favorite paddle, an ordeal-seeker is unlikely to let you know if things get to be too much: doing so feels to such a person like an admission that she has "failed." Make it clear to your partner that, for both of your safety, she *must* tell you if she feels that the spanking is damaging her physically or emotionally, and that nobody will consider that a sign of weakness or failure. And then watch her extra-carefully for signs of physical or emotional damage anyway.

A final category of spanking "script" comes from the bottom who seeks *humiliation*. Such folks are more attuned to the emotional aspects of spanking than to the physical ones. The more you load up the spanking scene with symbols of the power imbalance between the two of you – embarrassing positions, humiliating costumes, scornful lectures, corner time, playing with urine and/or enemas, kissing the implement, thanking you for each stroke – the better they like it.

Humiliation bottoms are easy on the hand, but hard on the imagination: coming up with ways to keep *both* sets of cheeks nice and pink can be a challenge. It's also worth remembering that professional dominants report that the humiliation-lover is the client most likely to "turn on" them in anger. Humiliation play can resonate down into the deepest levels of someone's self-image. It requires extra-careful step-by-step negotiation, even down to discussion of each word used in a scolding, in order to keep the scene emotionally safe for the bottom and physically safe for the top.

What's in it for tops?
The rewards of topping are a bit less tangible than those of bottoming – after all, it's the bottom who gets all the sensory goodies.

Contrary to most people's image of a spanker as heartless, cruel and sadistic, the rewards of spanking often actually stem from a deep empathy: if you weren't empathizing with the bottom's sensations, you might as well whack a pillow, right? Thus, the top can vicariously experience many of the same rewards the bottom is enjoying. Even "contact endorphin highs" are far from unknown (I've walked away from doing a heavy spanking feeling high as a kite).

Spanking, like being spanked, also offers us the opportunity to express aspects of ourselves that aren't safe or acceptable to act out in the real world: the brute, the strict authority figure, the sadist, the interrogator, the captor. When we find that within the clear boundaries of the spanking scene these personae are not just accepted, but lusted after and loved, a tremendous sense of healing and wholeness can result.

A persona is an aspect of yourself that comes out in a particular circumstance – like a spanking scene, for example.

And let's face it: the sounds and sensations and sights of spanking someone – the whimpers and moans and cries, the writhing and wiggling and clenching, the skin turning rosy and warm – are very, very sexy. It's not really very surprising that so many people are erotically attuned to an activity that involves so many sexual cues (in fact, it's sort of surprising to me that there are people who *aren't*).

Spanking fantasies

I've discussed at length some of the deep emotional "scripts" that underlie most spanking play. These scripts are often acted out within the context of a story – a story that we keep in our own heads, which we call a fantasy, or a story that we act out with a partner, which we call a scene.

Some of the commonest spanking fantasies have to do with *age play*. In these, one or both partners, usually the bottom, acts the part of someone younger than he really is. An age play bottom may be a cuddly, dependent infant, a fractious toddler, a naughty schoolchild, a rebellious teenager, a fraternity or sorority pledge. An age play top may be a nice or mean Mommy or Daddy, a strict schoolteacher or governess, a gung-ho coach, a sadistic frat boy, or another child (come on, didn't you and the other kids play spanking games together?). Age games give us a chance to relive our childhoods in an environment of safety and love, with a very unchildlike opportunity for adult sexual fun afterwards. They require some special safeguards to make sure that one adult can speak to one another out of role when necessary, and to avoid triggering unexpected regressions to genuine childhood trauma (see the "Communications" chapter for more information on how to set up these safeguards).

Other spanking fantasies have to do with *discipline*. Although few of us would actually like to be involved with a Singaporean judicial-style caning, many of us have fantasies about punishing or being punished in such an environment. Prison strappings, military discipline, and other adult discipline situations also have their adherents, particularly among gay men. However, acting out such a fantasy doesn't mean that you get to overlook your partner's real needs for warmup, communication, and nurturing; if you can't find ways to build those things directly into the narrative of your scene, take breaks when you need them to make sure everyone's OK.

Some people like to spank or be spanked within the context of a *captivity* scene. The top in such a scene may be a "rapist," "kidnapper," "inquisitor," "interrogator," or whatever her taste runs to; the bottom is her helpless "victim." Topping in a captivity scene is a little bit like driving with one foot on the accelerator and the other on the brake: at the same time as you're working to appear cruel, heartless and sadistic, you're keeping a close eye on your partner for signs of genuine distress or overload. The same cautions apply to captivity scenes as to adult discipline scenes – don't get carried away with your roles, and check in with one another often.

And finally, many spanking fans do their thing within the context of *ownership.* The bottom is often a slave, or occasionally an animal such as a puppy or horse. The "owner" may be spanking the bottom for his own pleasure, or as a disciplinary measure ("*Bad* dog!"); underlying the spanking is the fantasy that the owner has the right to use his property in any way he sees fit. I don't have to tell you, of course, that this is the U.S. in the '90s, and that nobody has the "right" to spank another adult – ownership fantasies, like any other, require careful attention to the realities of consent and limits.

These are just a few of the commonest fantasies and scripts enjoyed by spankers and spankees the world over; I'm sure you've got a few tasty ones of your own. But maybe these will give you a few new ideas and a bit of insight into the ideas that your fertile mind has already conjured.

4 Anatomy of a Spankee

The butt is a tough part of the body. It's mostly fat and muscle, with most of its bones and major nerves buried pretty deeply. Nevertheless, it's a good idea to know enough about its anatomy to avoid doing damage, and to focus on the most pleasurable spots.

You can refer to the drawing on page 19 to follow this section.

Opposite: If your paddle were an X-ray machine...

Starting from the inside, the **bones** of the butt are mostly the pelvis and the femurs (thigh bones), which are all large, sturdy bones. Unless you are spanking someone extremely elderly, you don't need to worry about injuring the pelvis or femur.

However, the butt also covers the lower end of the spine – the coccyx (COK-six), or tailbone. The tailbone tapers off approximately one-fourth to one-third of the way down the crack of the butt. It is relatively fragile, and quite sensitive to pain. A hard blow to the tailbone can cause damage which may require medical intervention to heal. It also feels extremely unpleasant and non-erotic to almost everybody. Therefore, before you spank someone hard (particularly with a heavy implement like a paddle), use your fingers to locate the end of their tailbone, and/or have them show you where it is. It may not be where you think it is: a fair number of tailbones get broken during childhood accidents and similar mishaps, so be sure you're feeling the right spot. (Your bottom should be able to tell you.) Avoid spanking on or near this spot.

Moving up through the tissues of the butt, the next area of concern is the **nerves**. The major nerve in the

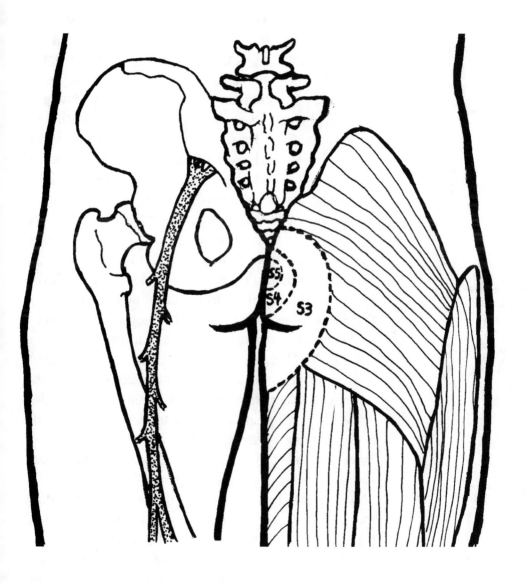

butt area is the sciatic nerve, which is the body's largest nerve. As you can see from the illustration, it starts at the pelvis and comes down the back of the thigh, buried deeply in the thigh muscles. Some cases are on record of long-term damage to the sciatic nerve from heavy paddling (usually in a fraternity hazing context). To avoid this injury, keep in mind that bent-over positions stretch and tighten the muscles of the butt and thigh, and thus offer less protection to the sciatic nerve. If you are going to hit hard with a spanking implement that is heavy in weight, it's a good idea to have your spankee either standing up or, better yet, lying face down. The heavier the implement and the harder the blow, the less bent-over he should be. (If you think he looks sexy bent over grabbing his ankles, stick to lighter, stingier implements.)

On a happier neurological note, take a look at the figure to see why so many of us get so turned on being spanked. The lower inner portion of the butt is fed by a nerve group called the "posterior S4 dermatome." If you had a similar map of the front of the body, you'd see that the S4 dermatome is shared by the genitals. Many spanking fans refer to this "low and inside" area as the "sweet spot," because being spanked there feels so good. A slightly broader area of the buttocks is fed by the posterior S3 dermatome, which also connects to the pubic area. Thus, smart spankers keep their "victims" coming back for more by focusing their attention on the lower inner quadrant of the buttocks. Of course, spanks can also be administered to other parts of the buttocks and upper thighs, but the smacks that keep your bottom moaning in that marvelous blend of ecstatic pain and pleasure are likely to be blows to the sweet spot.

When it comes to *muscles*, the majority of blows to the butt will land on the gluteus maximus, a large, strong muscle that covers the bulk of the buttock area. You may also land some blows on the long, heavy muscles of the upper and inner thigh. Most people of normal size and fitness have very strong muscles in this area, that do an excellent job of protecting underlying structures. If you are playing with a very thin or weak person, you might wish to stick to lighter, stingier toys, rather than heavy ones that might damage nerves or bones.

Avoid spanking above the top of the asscrack or below the midpoint of the thighs. About a hand-width above the bony protection of the pelvis, parallel to the elbows, lie the kidneys, which can be easily damaged by strong blows. The lower backs of the thighs and knees, where the thigh muscles thin out, contain relatively fragile tendons, ligaments and large blood vessels, and are too delicate to be struck in most people.

The *skin* of the butt is well fed with many small blood vessels. Many of the marks left by spanking result from damage to tiny capillaries (small blood vessels); the capillaries are broken and a small amount of blood is released under the skin. If your partner is taking any blood-thinning drug – which includes aspirin, ibuprofen, alcohol or coumadin – she will probably bruise more easily than usual. If it's important not to leave marks, avoid such drugs for 24 hours before play.

Some people find that the more they get spanked, the less likely they are to be marked.

Marks

While we're on the topic of marks, let's talk about some of the kinds of marks that can be left by a spanking. Mild spankings simply increase the circulation into the skin of the spanked area, turning it rosy and making it warm to the touch. This color usually fades away completely within an hour or two. Heavier spankings may cause the skin to raise up in a ridge or bump, usually pink or red in color, that we call a welt. Depending on the individual, welts may fade almost immediately, or may hang around for weeks. (Hot water from a shower or tub may bring a healed welt back up again – a fact learned to the embarrassment of one of my bottoms, who made the mistake of showering a week after our scene in the locker room of his branch of the armed forces!)

Some spankings may also leave bruises. Post-spanking bruising can range from a tiny darkened area through deep blackish-purple hematomas covering the entire buttock area. Bruising can take anywhere from a few days to several weeks to fade all the way from black to green to yellow to gone.

Some spankings, particularly those with rough-textured toys or toys with holes, can also blister or abrade the skin. Some people seem much more prone to this kind of injury than others; I've only experienced it twice in my career as a spankee. An abraded butt will look raw and oozy, and feel sticky to the touch. In extreme cases, it may even bleed. This type of mark takes the longest of all to heal, and may leave that part of the skin especially susceptible to future abrasion for a year or more.

For some people, any of the kinds of marks I've described here would cause a real problem. People who are in ostensibly monogamous relationships and people whose bodies are on display (such as dancers and models) have to be especially careful not to walk around marked. Some people who normally don't mind being marked have to be careful when they're scheduled an appointment with a doctor, chiropractor or bodyworker, or a trip to the beach or hot tub. Other people simply don't like the idea of wearing the evidence of their sexual predilections on their skin.

For help in finding health care practitioners who can deal with your spanking interest, check the Resource Guide.

Novice spankees tend to have very tender butts that often mark easily; experienced spankers sometimes develop skin which is tougher and thicker, so that they require more vigorous spankings to get where they want to go, and often tend not to mark easily. I've heard this condition called "leatherbutt" and "rhino butt." If your partner has a leather butt, he'll know it and tell you so. If he hasn't told you so, assume that he marks easily and behave accordingly.

I know people who have encountered <u>serious</u> problems in their relationships after showing up at home with unwanted (and unexpected) marks.

Never, ever promise anyone that you won't mark them – although it's certainly fine to promise to try your best to avoid it. It's impossible to know how easily someone marks if you've never played with them before. And people's markability varies from one session to the next, based on their health, their state of mind, what medications they're taking, and where (for women) they are in their menstrual cycle. However, a long slow warm-up so that everybody stays relaxed, plus a careful choice of toys, can help reduce the chances of marking. Spanking someone through their underwear can also reduce the chances of welts and abrasions, although it doesn't do much to prevent bruising.

If you're trying not to mark someone but do so anyway, take a look in the "Troubleshooting" chapter for some ideas for healing marks quickly.

If any mark has broken the skin – which means that if any sign of oozing or bleeding is present, no matter how small – it is important that you clean the toy extremely well before using it on anyone else, or, better yet, that you set the toy aside for use on that bottom only. The same rule applies if the toy has gotten semen, vaginal fluid or feces on it. AIDS, hepatitis and other diseases can be spread by carelessly using a contaminated toy on another bottom. See Appendix B for some techniques for cleaning spanking toys.

5 Communication and Mood

S ome of the most important time of your spanking scene takes place before a single pair of pants gets lowered. Talking straightforwardly about what kinds of activities interest you, about your desires and limits, is an essential part of making your spanking work. Without this negotiation process, tops are put in the awkward position of having to read bottoms' minds, and bottoms spend the entire spanking tense and on edge, wondering if the top is about to do something that the bottom really doesn't like. Hardly a formula for a successful interaction!

Many people aren't used to talking honestly about their erotic needs, so negotiation can be awkward if you're not used to it. It does get easier with practice – skilled negotiators can whiz through such conversations with dazzling ease.

Negotiation should be fun! Since when is talking dirty a chore?

I suggest that you and your partner have this discussion well before you get together to do your spanking scene. By the time you get together and are feeling all hot and bothered, your eagerness may lead you into making compromises that aren't a good idea. It's much easier to say "No, thanks," to a spanking that hasn't been planned yet than it is to walk away from an imminent scene.

Here are some of the topics you should probably discuss:

✥ The spanking itself. Hands only? Implements? Which implements are OK, which are to be used with caution, which are off limits? Any parts of the butt that don't like to be hit? Is it OK to hit anywhere besides the butt and, if so, where? Will it cause any problems if the spanking marks the bottom's skin?

♨ Sex. Will the spanking include any sexual interaction? If so, what kind? What are both parties' standards for safer sex: which activities are safe enough to do without a barrier, which ones require a barrier, which are too unsafe to do at all? Who will be in charge of providing safer sex materials such as condoms, gloves and lubricant?

♨ Roles. Who will top, and who will bottom? Will the spanking include any role-playing such as teacher/student, owner/slave, parent/child or captor/captive?

For more detailed help with negotiation, check out some of the S/M books listed in the Resource Guide.

♨ Related activities. Will the spanking include any bondage, and, if so, in what positions and with what materials? Will other activities such as role-playing, humiliation games, or enemas be involved?

♨ Physical limits. Does either partner have any physical conditions that should be taken into account? Common physical limits include heart trouble, back trouble, easy bruising due to anemia or diabetes, breathing difficulty, seizure disorders, and circulatory problems.

♨ Emotional limits. Does either partner have any history of being nonconsensually abused or assaulted? If so, what activities might trigger unwanted memories of the abuse?

♨ Communication during the scene. How will you let each other know if something isn't working out right? Some suggestions follow.

Straightforward verbal communication

In all consensual erotic spanking scenes, from the most lovingly playful to the harshest, it is essential to maintain good ongoing communication and feedback between the top and the bottom. Getting or giving the information you need to, without interfering with whatever roles or fantasies you may be playing out, is one of the highest arts of any form of erotic power exchange.

Often, communication may take place in the simplest of verbal forms: "I'm getting a cramp in my thigh," "This is scaring me – let's back off a bit," "Wait; did you hear someone in the hallway?" Such communications are clear and straightforward, and need not interfere more than momentarily in the scene: accomplished players get very fluid about stopping for a moment to take care of a problem, then dropping back into role almost immediately.

"One to ten"

When you're playing with a new bottom or with a new toy or technique, it can become important to "calibrate" the sensations – some bottoms are bored by spankings that would send other bottoms into traumatic hysteria. An excellent way for tops to gain information about a new sensation is called "one to ten." In this technique, the top delivers one extremely gentle stroke, hardly more than laying the implement onto the bottom's skin, and explains, "That was a 'one' on a scale of one to ten. 'Ten' would be the hardest I'm willing to hit you. For the next few minutes, I want you to use that number scale to tell me how hard a stroke you want to feel. I won't hit you anyplace but on your butt, and I won't hit you until you tell me to." After a few minutes of this type of communication, the top has some idea of the bottom's desires, and the bottom has had a chance to relax into the idea of being spanked. Both partners can decide together when it's time to stop one-to-tenning and to turn over more control to the top.

Safewords

When spankees like to pretend that we're not consenting to this terrible, horrible, awful thing that's happening to us, communication can become tricky. Many if not most spankophiles have fantasies of nonconsent, and enjoy expressing ourselves in that fashion – and it can be very difficult for a top to know exactly what you mean by your ecstatic shrieks of "No! Please! Stop!"

Thus was born the "safeword." One of the key tools in helping to keep spanking play physically and emotionally safe for all concerned, a safeword is simply a code word that means "Something about this *really* isn't working for me, and we need to stop and talk about it." Many players have two safewords – one that means "Slow down for a second and give me a chance to talk; there's something I need to tell you" and a second that means "Stop this scene right now; something is seriously wrong." Here on the West Coast, these are often "yellow" and "red," but you can use whatever words you like as long as they're easy for both players to remember and pronounce.

I've heard that in Chicago they use "411" for "information" and "911" for "emergency."

Although people tend to think of safewords as something that bottoms use when a sensation becomes too intense, my experience with them is that they're really used that way less often than you might think. They tend to come up when someone in the scene is having a physical or emotional problem, which may or may not be related to the spanking itself – illness, recognition of a real-world problem ("Oh my God, I was supposed to be home a half hour ago!"), or awareness of physical or emotional danger. Tops can and do safeword too, if something in the scene becomes too intense or difficult for them.

Some players resent the idea of safewords, feeling that they give the bottom too much control over what's going on. My belief is that, in a consensual scene, there are always safewords – verbal or physical cues that the bottom can use to say "Stop this right now." Since I think "red" is politer than "take your frigging hands off me or I'm calling the cops," I prefer to use prenegotiated safewords. (If you don't enjoy role-playing nonconsent, then you may choose to use everyday language instead. This is fine. My point is simply that communications in spanking scenes need to be clear and unambiguous.)

My partner Jay Wiseman introduced this technique in his book "SM 101: A Realistic Introduction." It works very well.

opposite: *This position offers much of the same physical contact as over-the-knee, but may be more comfortable for both top and bottom.*

In some cases, a bottom cannot safeword for some reason – sometimes because he has a gag in his mouth, sometimes because he's gone into a deeply emotional, non-verbal state, and has forgotten the whole concept. Many players have developed some sort of gesture they can use as a safeword equivalent. One popular one is the "two squeezes" technique: the top takes hold of some part of the bottom's body – preferably not one of the parts she's been playing with – and gives it two firm squeezes, which asks the bottom, "Are you OK with what's going on?" The bottom gives some part of the top's body two squeezes in response. If the response is not forthcoming, the top repeats the "question"; if the bottom is still unresponsive, it's time to stop the scene and communicate verbally. I've talked to other players who have evolved other nonverbal codes such as "thumbs up/thumbs down," or giving the bottom some sort of noisemaking device like a clicker or squeaky toy, which she can squeeze to alert her top if she gets into trouble. Any of these can work, as long as each of you understands what the other's signals mean.

Role-playing

One of the trickiest parts of communicating during spanking play is maintaining appropriate dialogue and mood. If you enjoy spanking as sensuous foreplay only, you may not choose to explore this kind of fantasy play. But if you have fantasies of being a child and a punitive teacher, or a slave and a demanding master, or a puppy and a scolding owner, a certain amount of theater will help keep the fantasy alive.

However, many players find this kind of role-playing difficult, making them feel self-conscious and "silly." How can you get past that awkwardness to create the scenes you enjoy?

One good guideline to keep in mind is to keep it simple. As a human being, you are blessed with the gift

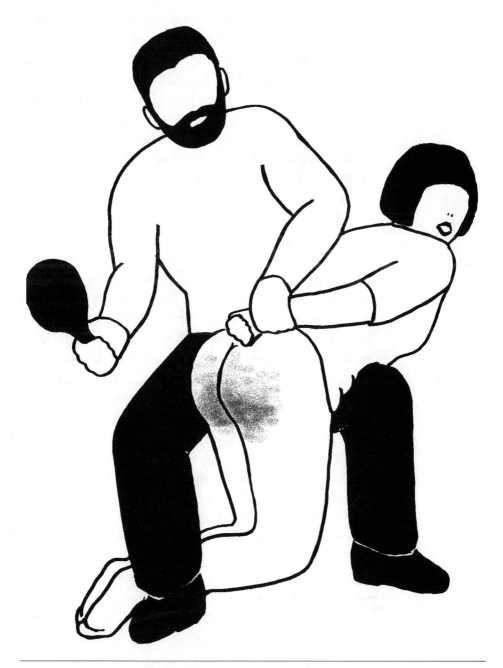

of imagination: you don't need an entire pirate movie set, complete with ship; perhaps a genteelly evil partner with a ruffled shirt, plus a few convincing lines of dialogue, will do the trick.

Many spanking devotees are strongly eroticized to certain key words or phrases: the word "spanking" itself, descriptions like "naughty," appellations like "young lady," directions like "get those trousers down," or predictions like "you won't sit down for a week" get many, many people's juices flowing. Clever tops watch their bottoms for a sudden blush or quickening of the breath when such phrases are used. Likewise, bottoms often enjoy turning on their tops with a judicious bit of "sincere" pleading or whimpering.

One of the secrets of role-playing is that the more aroused you are, the more natural the role seems. In the beginning of the scene, when both of you are a little self-conscious and not yet turned on, such dialogue may seem awkward. I recommend that you say it anyway, and say it as convincingly as you can: I can almost guarantee that a nice surge of hardness or wetness – your own and your partner's – will reward your efforts. As you get more turned on, the phrases will seem less and less silly, and more and more arousing, until you're both in full (so to speak) swing.

Those who like their scenes theatrical may enjoy experimenting with props and costumes – many a spankophile was elated by the recent fashion trend toward schoolgirl-style pleated skirts and knee socks for adults. If you enjoy that kind of thing and have the time and money for thrift-store excursions, go for it. But even if you don't, a little mental scene-setting, combined with imaginative dialogue well-spiced with time-honored spanking phrases, will get your scene off and running.

6 Warmup

E ven the greediest masochist is unlikely to have a good time if you start a scene with half a dozen heavy strokes from The Cane From Hell. To take your bottom to bliss, you have to start slowly, with a nice warmup – bringing up his circulation, letting his endorphins rev up, helping him relax into the sensation.

I've seen tops linger for as much as an hour over warmup, starting with gentle caresses, escalating slowly to little pats, then to light smacks, then to harder spanks... progressing to the intense stuff only when the bottoms are so thoroughly blissed out that they're pushing their backsides out to meet the paddle, and laughing ecstatically as the strokes fall.

For certain types of scenes, such as punishment scenes, you may wish to skip warmup, deliberately making it difficult for your bottom to process and enjoy the pain. I recommend that you try this only with a bottom you know very well and have played with often. If you do try it, expect your bottom to mark much more easily than usual, and be prepared for a strong emotional reaction of anger or sadness.

In general, however, I strongly recommend as much warmup as your patience and arm can accommodate. Few bottoms mind a slow-building warmup, and for many, it's essential. If your bottom is at all tense or nervous, or if it's been a long time since she's last played, take some extra time during warmup.

Remember, warmup is for tops too – it's a time to get in touch with your bottom, to limber up your own arm and shoulder to help prevent injuries, to get yourself into role, to establish the rhythm and flow of the scene. A warmup is to spanking what foreplay is to sex: don't rush it!

7 Implements

So you've got your bottom warmed up and panting for more. How do you keep up the good work? Part of your decision-making process may have to do with choosing and using spanking implements.

Choosing and Using Implements

Responsible tops don't use a toy on anybody else unless they've felt it on their own bodies. At minimum, give yourself several good sharp blows with a potential toy in a well-padded spot such as your upper back, thigh or butt. Better yet, have a trusted friend give you a few swats. This kind of precaution does not in any way diminish your authority as a top; it enhances it – you're not just a mean sonovabitch, you're a *careful* mean sonovabitch.

You often hear spanking toys ranked on a spectrum ranging from "sting" to "thud." Stingy toys are felt mostly on the skin, with a sharp sensation; thuddy toys echo down into deeper structures of muscle and even bone. As a general rule, the heavier a toy is in proportion to its breadth, the thuddier it is. Stingy toys tend to leave welts and, with extreme use, can cut skin; thuddy toys tend to leave bruises and can, with extreme use, cause damage to nerves and bones. Many bottoms have marked preferences for either sting or thud – which does not, of course, mean that you have to give them only the kinds of sensations they like, unless their preference is strong enough to be expressed as a definite limit.

Aim is important. I always enjoy looking at the aftermath of a spanking administered by a knowledgeable and experienced spanker: the rosy color is nicely concentrated in the sweet spot, with just enough pinkness spread around other parts of the butt area to let you know that the top wasn't *too* overly concerned with her bottom's pleasure only.

This kind of control is easy with a hand, and only slightly harder with a short, inflexible implement like a hairbrush. But how do you achieve such attractive results with toys that are long, floppy, or otherwise unwieldy? To explain, I need to talk a bit about the physics of spanking implements.

Imagine the arc of, say, a strap, as it swings through the air, about to crack over a helpless backside. The part of the strap held in the hand is moving as fast as the hand itself. But the free end of the strap is traveling through a much larger arc, and is thus moving much faster. It is this tip that will strike the skin with the greatest force.

Many novice spankers make the mistake of aiming the center of their spanking tool at the area they wish to strike. The center of our imaginary strap might thus fall quite nicely on the lower center of the recipient's buttock. Meanwhile, however, that vicious tip is following through and executing an agonizing one-point landing way over on the far hip. This phenomenon is called "wrapping."

Everybody wraps occasionally; a few tops do it on purpose (a particularly nasty trick is to aim for the center of a thigh so that the tip of your implement wraps around and bites the inner thighflesh). But more than one or two unintentional welts on hips or outer thighs is a sure sign of a top whose ambitions exceed his expertise.

The cure for wrapping is a combination of practice and feedback. Tops: Before you use an instrument that is the least bit floppy or whippy on actual flesh, practice on an inanimate object such as a cushion, quilt or plush toy. (Yes, you may feel silly beating the snot out of Teddy, but that's better than feeling sillier when your bottom walks away from you with marks in places where they shouldn't

I like to practice on a quilt, aiming the tip of my toy for the place where the stitching intersects.

It's not too rare for a top to get so caught up in the role that she forgets the need to communicate honestly and politely. It's important to discuss this – preferably outside scene space – to make sure that everybody is able to get their needs met.

be.) Bottoms: A top who's wrapping probably doesn't know it. *Politely* telling her that a stroke or two has wrapped, using whatever type of communication the two of you have established, is an important form of feedback for her, and will enable her to do her job better. (A top who chides you for giving polite and honest factual feedback during a scene is a top to re-educate or avoid.)

With long or flexible toys, it's a good idea to learn to spank from both directions, so that the heaviest part of the spanking gets well distributed onto both cheeks. If the bottom is lying face down and you're moving around, this is simple: just walk from one side of the bed or table to the other. If she's standing up, you'll have to either learn to strike with your non-dominant hand, or develop your backhand. Either of these techniques may take a bit more practice than you used for your regular stroke, but will be well worth it.

Hands

While spankophiles are often avid collectors of paddles, straps, canes and the like – I know a few who own thousands of dollars' worth – the fact is that you need no equipment at all to perform an extremely enjoyable and effective spanking.

Even if you've got a steamer trunk full of gear, I strongly recommend that you start your spankings with your hand. Handspankings offer a greater range of sensation than any implement ever could: gentle loving caresses, warm sensuous smacks, harsh stinging slaps, deep thuddy jolts. Moreover, spanking someone with your hand offers a tremendous amount of feedback. You get a much clearer idea of exactly what each spank feels like to your bottom, since the sensation is echoed into your hand.

Many spanking aficionadoes enjoy only hand-spanking, and are frightened or offended by the use of

*A handspanking
isn't necessarily a
light spanking.
Some spankers
have hands of iron
that hurt a lot,
bless their hearts.*

implements for spanking. That's fine – a skilled spanking hand is like a bag of toys at the end of your arm.

You can spank with fingers only, with the palm, or with the heel of your hand; with the hand flat or cupped; with a glancing blow that slides along the skin, or a straight-on smack; with a "popping" motion that snatches the hand away from the skin almost on contact, or with deep follow-through; with many quick little smacks covering wide areas, or with slow, hard spanks with long pauses between. Experiment with keeping your hand and wrist rigid, or leaving them floppy. What does it feel like when your fingers are held tightly together, or spread loosely apart? Try drumming with two hands, like you would on bongo drums... using the heel of your hand to deliver a heavy jolting blow upwards against the base of the butt... alternating hard strokes with caresses to keep your bottom off-balance and guessing.

It might be fun and educational to do a session or two in which you and your bottom experiment with these and other strokes, asking her to give you lots of feedback about how each one feels.

One word of warning: if you're like me – a tender-handed person who plays with tough-butted bottoms – you may find that handspanking may all too literally "hurt you more than it does them." Gloves can help. A close-fitting latex, vinyl, or lightweight leather glove can take some of the sting out of your hand and put it into their backside where it belongs. Padded motorcyclists' gloves can help protect your hand from very heavy spanking blows. Also, many spankees enjoy the contrasting sensations available from a lace or fishnet glove, or a fingerless glove. Experiment!

Paddles

I am using the term "paddles" to cover the entire range of spanking implements that are broad, stiff and flat. Paddles range from fairly tame implements of stiffened leather through large, heavy wooden boards. Their sensation may be quite stingy – plastic paddles are often viciously so – or may thud down into muscle and bone.

Many people who have tried and enjoyed handspanking decide that the next logical step is to use a hairbrush, which is basically a small paddle. Be careful with this: hairbrushes are nastier than many people realize. They concentrate the full force of a spanking blow into a small, hard area, so they hurt a lot, and they're likely to leave bruises. (One of my favorite spankees, an avid masochist who hugely enjoys intense floggings and canings, refuses to have a hairbrush used on her.)

To my mind, the logical next step up from handspanking is a well-crafted leather paddle. These are available in any leather store and most erotic boutiques, or if you are handy with tools you can make your own from stiff leather. An implement called a "slapper," basically a flexible, double-thick leather paddle in which the paddle ends are left unattached so that they smack together upon impact, is available in riding supply stores at a very reasonable cost, and also makes an excellent first paddle.

Perhaps more than any other spanking toy, paddles can be found in all sorts of environments. Paddles from games such as ping-pong can serve very well (a lawn game called Jokari includes large, round, plywood paddles that have something of a cult following). Housewares stores often sell big, solid wooden spoons, as well as wooden and plastic cheeseboards which make good heavy paddles. Thrift stores and antique stores sometimes yield novelty paddles with corny sayings on them ("Board of Education" and the like), as well as authentic fraternity paddles. One of my favorite paddles is the rubber sole of a discarded martial arts shoe. Once you start looking around, you'll begin to feel like you're surrounded by paddles.

It can be fun to tease freshly spanked skin by running the bristles of the hairbrush over it, though.

When buying a paddle designed for another use, be sure it's strong and smooth enough to be used for spanking.

Some paddles have holes in them; devotees claim that the holes diminish wind resistance, enabling the spanker to strike harder. While I have my doubts about that, there is no question that paddles with holes are stingier and likelier to blister or abrade skin. The holes also create structural weakness in the paddle, so that these paddles are likelier than others to break.

In acquiring a paddle, look for a smooth, cleanly finished surface, with nicely beveled or rounded edges and corners – sharp edges are likely to cause damage. If the paddle is designed for striking, such as a game paddle or a paddle made especially for spanking, it's unlikely to break unless used quite hard. If you're using something designed for another purpose, check it frequently during the spanking to make sure it hasn't cracked or broken.

Many paddles – even those made for the purpose – are, in my opinion, a bit large for good spanking play. If you're spanking with a large paddle, particularly if your partner has a small butt, you can hardly avoid hitting over and over again on the same spot. I prefer a slightly smaller paddle that I can keep moving over the entire area.

In our household we call this the "wuss paddle" and use it as a penalty for Truth Or Dare games.

A special subtype of paddle is perfect for situations in which one or both partners like the idea of a paddling, but the bottom doesn't enjoy the sensation of pain. If you find yourself in such a situation, the foam rubber "kneeling pads" sold in garden supply stores are a great solution: you can swing them as hard as you can, they make an incredibly loud "whack," and they feel like a mild tap on the bottom's behind. You can role-play as fierce a beating as you like without causing your bottom a moment's physical discomfort.

Straps

For the sake of simplicity, I'll refer to any spanking implement that's long, narrow and very flexible as a strap.

Many bottoms absolutely love to be struck with a strap. On the other hand, a fair number of people have been nonconsensually beaten with straps as children, so these toys may have a stronger chance than other implements of awakening buried memories or strong emotions. In order to avoid such occurrences, I recommend that you negotiate the use of a strap before you haul one out and start flailing away.

The classic strap, of course, is the top's belt, and the sound of a belt being tugged out of its loops sends a special shiver down many bottoms' spines. If you enjoy this sort of thing, it's worth acquiring one or two belts especially for spanking games. Look for belts of supple leather, at least an inch and a half wide, with no harsh stitching or metal parts on the striking area. If you have, or can find, an old, wide, well-worn leather belt from the '60s or '70s, you've got a spanking treasure: recondition it, if necessary,

I use Dr. Jackson's Hide Rejuvenator from Tandy Leather.

with a good hide rejuvenator, and look forward to making some bottom very happy.

Other straps can be found in riding supply stores – my favorite strap is a wide leather cinch strap from a saddle. Old razor strops can often be found in antique stores; cut away the canvas backing and you've got a wonderful strap. Straps of leather or rubber (watch out for the latter; rubber is nastier than you might expect) are also a good do-it-yourself project.

Straps are especially likely to wrap. Many straps made for non-spanking purposes contribute to this problem by being a bit too long for the average butt. To compensate, fold the strap in half and hold the loose ends in your hand, striking with the doubled-up part; or simply wrap part of the strap around your hand and use the remainder to strike with. (Please don't ever try to strike anyone with the buckle or metallic parts of a belt. You can lacerate their skin deeply that way.) If you acquire a

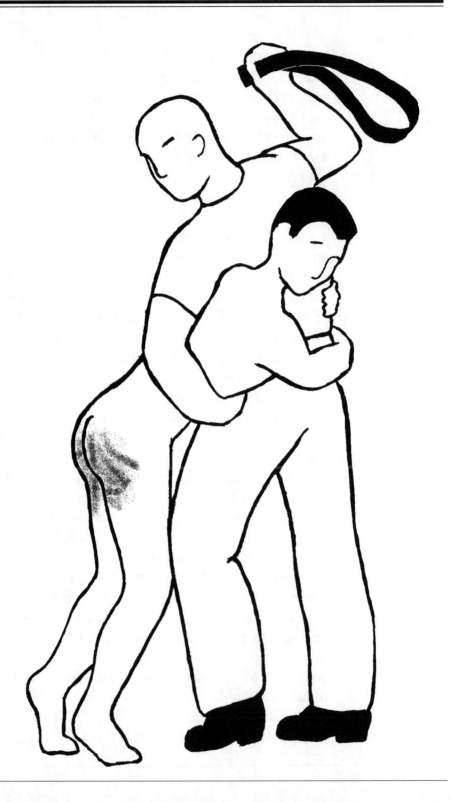

new strap, practice on something inanimate before you try using it on a person.

Birch Rods

The birch rod, sometimes called just the birch, has a long and honorable history. Although it is seldom used punitively today, it played a significant role in the Victorian schoolroom and in many prisons in earlier centuries.

The birch consists of six to 12 long, thin, whippy branches cut from a birch or similar tree, with the twigs and, if possible, the buds left on. The branches are tied together at the thick end with string or ribbon, and left splaying out at the thin end. A good birch should be broad enough to spread out over a good part of the butt with each stroke, and should be dense enough to bite in many places at once without being so dense as to feel like a broom. If you have access to a birch tree, they are easy to make (be sure and rinse the branches well to remove dust, dirt and smog). During a birching, little bits of birch twig and bark tend to break loose and fly all over the place; you can minimize this phenomenon by soaking your birch in water for eight or so hours beforehand, but you should still expect to do some sweeping or vacuuming afterewards.

left: the underarm position, with a belt.

Being birched feels like being stung simultaneously by an entire swarm of angry insects. It marks the butt with hundreds of little crisscrossed lines, often intersected by small dark spots where the buds bit into the skin. It is likelier than most other forms of spanking to abrade or break the skin, so it's important to use each birch rod on only one bottom.

Floggers and Other Multi-Tailed Implements

Many spankophiles enjoy playing with multi-tailed flagellation implements, usually made of leather but sometimes of other materials – floggers, flails, cats-o-nine-tails, and the like. While instructions for truly skilled use of these toys could fill their own book, a few notes here can at least get you started.

Floggers can deliver sensations ranging from the most sensuous of massage-like caresses through skin-tearing agony. If you're considering the purchase of your first flogger, don't make the mistake many novice tops do (I speak from experience here) – don't buy the biggest, nastiest, meanest-looking flogger you can find. Using a flogger well takes a lot of practice, and you want to start with an implement that forgives your mistakes: try a flogger of soft suede, deerskin, or a similar material. Such floggers are ideal for warmup, and excellent for many other kinds of spanking as well. Save floggers of heavy leather, and braided or knotted floggers, for later if ever.

When I'm flogging a woman who is face down, I especially like to stand at her head and flog her "sweet spot" so that some of the tails of the flogger land on her pussy.

Floggers do not work well in positions that bring the top's body very close to the bottom's, such as over-the-knee spanking. On the other hand, they can be used very effectively on a standing bottom or on one who is lying face down.

Most people start out with a simple side stroke: if you're right-handed and your bottom is standing, stand to his left side and bring the flogger around so that its tips land in the center of his right cheek. Once you get comfortable with that, you can add more strokes to your repertoire, such as a backhand stroke, a figure-eight, a twirling stroke and more. (People who are really into floggers often look like they're performing some specialized rhythmic gymnastics routine.)

Floggers are perhaps the likeliest of all common spanking toys to cause problems with wrapping. Put in some serious practice on an inanimate object before you use one on a human being.

Many spanking folks think of floggers as being more about traditional S/M than about spanking. But skilled and judicious use of a flogger can, if you like it, add a delightful dimension to many spanking scenes.

Canes, Crops, Switches and the Like

Long, narrow, fairly rigid implements offer what is probably the most intense sensation available to the spanking enthusiast. For this reason, they require particular care and skill to use safely.

Few U.S. residents have ever seen or felt a whipping cane; however, they are still in use in many scholastic and judicial environments in other parts of the world. The cane typically used by spanking enthusiasts is modeled on the canes used in British public schools over the last couple of centuries – not on the much heavier, longer, more brutal implements used on criminals in some African and Asian nations.

Canes used for spanking play are usually made of rattan or, occasionally, of manmade materials such as fiberglass or Delrin. (Bamboo is generally considered unsuitable for canes, due to its tendency to split lengthwise, leaving a knifelike edge. You can tell the difference between bamboo and rattan by examining the joints: the joints in rattan look like a telescope, with each section slightly smaller than the last one. Bamboo joints form a ridge without any telescope effect.)

Most canes used in spanking play are about three to three and a half feet long, and range in diameter from a quarter inch to a bit less than half an inch. A well-made cane has all its edges carefully sanded, with a nice rounded end and no sharp or harsh places at the joints. Opinions vary about whether canes should be varnished or not; I prefer mine varnished. Don't worry if your rattan cane isn't perfectly straight – since rattan is an organic material, it tends to curve slightly. You can minimize the curvature by storing your cane flat or hanging, instead of propping it against a wall. The holding end may be left plain, rounded into a crook, or finished with a handle of leather or another material.

Canes are flexible but not floppy. (They do wrap, although not as much as straps or floggers.) They should bend into a shallow C shape under pressure, but are not typically flexible enough to be bent entirely in half. To maintain flexibility in a rattan cane, you will have to soak it occasionally. If it's varnished, sand the varnish off the tip, then place the cane tip down in a bowl, cup or tub of water overnight. Let it dry and then, if desired, re-varnish the tip with a couple of coats of marine spar varnish.

Canes that aren't soaked regularly tend to get brittle.

Canes can be applied with a series of brisk, sharp taps all over the butt, which provides a glowing sting all over the skin. Or they can be administered with a sharp, wristy stroke which most bottoms find intensely painful (although many absolutely love it for that reason). Hard cane strokes leave a unique two-tracked mark that may last quite a while. Too many of them, particularly from a thin whippy cane, will break the skin.

The sensation of a cane is a bit different from that of most spanking implements. It arrives in two waves: a sharp jolt upon impact, followed by a rushing wave of pain a moment later. It is considerate to allow your bottom enough time to process that second wave of pain (if you watch closely, you may actually be able to see the sensation move through his body) before you administer another stroke. On the other hand, if you're feeling mean, administering several sharp cane strokes without much time between them can challenge the abilities of even a very talented masochist.

Riding crops are a twofold implement. You can use the tip only, as a small paddle, delivering a rain of quick little blows all over the butt. Or you can use the shaft like a heavy cane. In either case, it's important to choose your crop carefully. Crops intended for use as a paddle should have broad, stiffish, flexible tips. If you want to strike with the shaft, examine the crop carefully for harsh stitching that could cause problems, and take an extra-careful look at how the tip is attached to the shaft: many crops use stiff wire-like wrapping that hurts in a very non-erotic way and can easily cause more damage than you intended.

A third sort of cane-type implement is a switch – a slim, flexible branch cut from a tree. The severity of switches depends strongly on the type of tree, size and greenness of branch, and so on; the most severe can cause more damage than most spankees are comfortable with, so start out slowly with any new switch. Since switches can break skin, make sure you haven't cut yours from any kind of toxic plant like an oleander. A traditional old-fashioned preamble to punishment was to send the miscreant out to the yard to cut his own switch; if you have a yard with trees, give it a try yourself.

8 Positions

T he choice of position has a significant impact on the flavor and tone of your spanking scene. Some positions put the bottom's body under stress, creating tension and intensity; others enable the bottom to relax, promoting a "floaty," ecstatic scene.

In choosing positions, it's important to take into consideration your bottom's build, state of health, and preferences, as well as your own: the over-the-knee position that sends a large top and tiny bottom rocketing into bliss may be impractical, absurd or even dangerous for a tiny woman who wants to spank a large, heavy man.

For the purposes of categorization, I'm going to break spanking positions into two categories: upright and face-down. Each category, as you'll see, has many variations.

Upright Positions

This category includes any position in which most of the bottom's weight is borne by her feet.

The most basic upright position is *standing*, in which the bottom is simply standing up, without support. This is a simple position which can be used in any environment. Gravity tends to pull the bottom's butt muscles downward a bit, so you may want to hit a little lower than usual. Hard spanks may create problems in balance for the bottom; a considerate top either allows her to brace her hands against a sturdy wall or piece of furniture, or steadies her with the non-spanking hand.

Standing positions often work out quite well. For very heavy spanking scenes, the bottom might find that the effort of maintaining balance is distracting him from the spanking. Also, he may have trouble holding still in this position. Still, standing positions are suitable for bottoms of most body types and styles.

Those who like to combine bondage with their spanking often enjoy tying the bottom's wrists together and fastening them to an overhead attachment point. If bondage of this or any other kind interests you, take a look at Appendix C for a few pointers.

A more challenging upright position is **bent over.** Bent-over positions are very erotic for many spankers and spankees, and have a place in most spanking fans' repertoires. However, it's worth keeping in mind that bending over stretches out the muscles of the butt and thighs, and thus makes blows feel more harsh and intense than they might otherwise seem. Keeping someone bent over for a long period of time can also impair her breathing and circulation, increasing the likelihood of discomfort, panic or even fainting.

If you're spanking a bent-over male, watch out for his testicles! To protect these delicate organs – which could be seriously damaged by a hard blow – shield them with your non-dominant hand, have him keep his legs closed, or have him protect them himself with his own hands. Some men like to wear a leather g-string as additional protection. Such safeguards are particularly important if you're using an implement that is long, floppy or unwieldy, such as a strap, cane or flogger.

Many tops enjoy the sight of a bottom bent fully over and **grabbing her ankles**, the position often imposed by headmasters with canes in England and coaches with paddles in the U.S. However, for those of us who are perhaps not as young and slim as the average schoolchild, this position can be difficult to attain and even harder to hold. Hard blows to someone in this position can also knock them dangerously off-balance.

See illustration on
p. 77.

The ***head-between-legs*** position is a variation on the bent-over position that solves some of these problems. In this variation, the spankee bends over as though he were going to grab his ankles. Then, however, the spanker stands in front of him with her legs spread slightly and with his head between her legs. The bottom grabs the top's legs for balance. While a very tall top might have trouble reaching the sweet spot on the butt of a very short bottom, and while an overweight or out-of-shape bottom might have trouble bending over this far, this position works nicely for many people.

See illustration on
p. 40.

Another good bent-over position, the ***underarm*** position, works best with largish tops and smallish bottoms. The bottom bends over and the top stands beside her, grasping her around the waist with his non-dominant arm. The dominant hand is thus left free for its painful tasks.

See illustration on
p. 68.

Midway between the upright positions and the face-down positions are positions in which the bottom is ***bent over an object*** such as a table, chair or bed, thus taking the weight of the upper body on the object while keeping the weight of the lower body on the feet. This position is comfortable for most bottoms and can be held for a longer period of time than many others. It combines well with bondage if you're so inclined, and can be executed in almost any environment, from a dungeon to a guest bedroom. This is certainly one of the most popular spanking positions, and deservedly so. A pillow under the bottom's chest may help protect the neck from uncomfortable strain.

Face-Down Positions

In this category I include all positions in which most of the bottom's weight rests on the front of the body.

The classic spanking position is, of course, ***over the knee.*** (Since people reading this book are of adult stature, it might be more accurate to say "over the lap" – most grown-ups take up more space than a single knee can provide. Still, the phrase, often abbreviated to "OTK," is well established.)

See illustration on p. 8.

Over-the-knee spanking is beloved by many and plays a central role in many spankophiles' fantasies. If the spankee is relatively lightweight and fit, the classic OTK position may work out quite well. However, larger spankees, or those who are a bit overweight or inflexible, may have trouble holding this position for any length of time – it may impair their breathing or cause an uncomfortable amount of stress in their arms and legs. Small-lapped tops might also have trouble with this position (it's not much fun spanking someone when your legs have gone numb).

A couple of variations can help solve these problems. The first is for the spanker to seat himself on a **bed or couch**, enabling the bottom to stretch out across his lap, with chest and legs supported by the surface. If you plan to hold this position for long, make sure there is sufficient support – a headboard or couch back – for the top's back.

A second variation is to adapt the classic OTK position by having the top sit on a very **short stool or chair**. Because the bottom is closer to the floor, he can take some of his weight on his hands and feet or knees, thus reducing pressure on his abdomen and on his top's legs. If you are fond of over-the-knee spanking, a small stool such as those sometimes sold for children (make sure it can bear both of your weight) can be an excellent investment.

See illustration on p. 48.

Or you can try shifting the bottom's position relative to the top in a couple of ways, while still maintaining that mildly humiliating OTK energy so beloved of many tops and bottoms. Have her kneel between the top's legs, bending over one knee. Or she can even try taking a wheelbarrow-like position, with her hands on the floor between his feet and her legs spread to either side of his waist, so her butt points up towards his face.

A second form of face-down position is to have the bottom *lie on her stomach* on a bed or sturdy table. Adding a few pillows under her hips may make this position more comfortable and will definitely present her butt at an inviting angle. (If you have one of those backrests shaped like the arms and back of a chair, try turning it face-down and using it under her hips.) Some bottoms may also require a pillow under their chests in order to reduce strain on their necks. This is probably the most comfortable, relaxed position of all for most bottoms.

Spankees can also be placed on *all fours*, either on a surface or on the floor. This position can be fun for a while, but will tire most bottoms' wrists and arms out fairly quickly.

See illustration on p. 86.

The *knees-and-chest* position, in which the bottom kneels down and then lowers his chest to the floor so his butt sticks up in the air, has a great deal to recommend it. The arms can be stretched beyond his head (yoga practitioners will recognize this as "child pose"), crossed under his head to cushion and brace his head and neck, or you can have him lace his fingers together behind his neck. This is a very attractive position which offers terrific access to the butt; many tops are very aroused by the sight of the protruding backside as it jerks, twitches, clenches and squirms. Some bottoms, however, may find this position stressful on their backs, necks or knees. Allowing the bottom to spread his knees, or placing a small pillow under the fronts of his ankles, may help.

Many spanking fans sooner or later find themselves thinking about designing and constructing a *spanking bench*. While designs for these delightful toys vary widely, they are all basically designed to hold the bottom's body in a bent-over or all-fours position, with or without bondage. The best spanking benches I've seen include adjustable arm and leg rests so that the bench can be configured for different bodies, and plenty of padding under the spankee's chest and abdomen. I've seen benches shaped like well-padded sawhorses, benches shaped like half-barrels, benches shaped like vaulting horses, and several other models. Designs for spanking benches can be seen in some S/M and spanking books and magazines as well as in professional dungeons and play spaces; if you're considering buying or building one, check out several different designs – playing on them if possible – to see which ones you like best.

9 Afterwards

So it's all over, and it was great. Your arm is almost as sore as your bottom's butt, and you're both breathing hard, excited and happy and satisfied.

Although you don't often read about it in spanking porn, the time *after* the spanking is one of the most important parts of your play. A good spanking scene creates its own reality – a reality of intimate connection, of lowered boundaries and tremendous intimacy. Learning to cherish and prolong that reality is one of the high arts of spanking.

At a bare minimum, it's a good idea to spend a while cuddling and nurturing each other. Bottoms need support and nurturance as they emerge from the vulnerable space of the spanking back into everyday reality. Tops may also need support – although many people fail to realize it, administering a spanking can be scary and guilt-inducing, and it's a wise bottom who spends lots of time letting her top know how much she enjoyed herself and how grateful she is.

If you and your partner have agreed to have sex as part of your spanking scene, now is the time. You may feel like launching directly into hot and heavy fucking, or you may need some time of gentleness and quiet before you're ready to begin building sexual energy. Be sensitive to one another's cues in this area, and if your partner seems to be misreading you, it's fine to politely say so and ask for a little more – or less – recovery time.

If you haven't agreed to be sexual, it's still a good idea to spend some time together. A meal or a drink, preferably in a kitchen or restaurant with nice soft seats, can be a very pleasant way to decompress after a spanking. Or you can watch some TV, take a shower together, play a game – anything that allows the two of you to come out of your own special reality and back into the "real" world in one another's company.

I don't suggest that you spend too much time right after the spanking talking about how you liked it or didn't like it, or what did or didn't work for you – the alternate reality of your spanking universe may still have a stronger grip on your mind and emotions than you realize. It's a very good idea, however, to check in with one another the next day, by phone or e-mail or, better yet, in person. During this conversation, you can compare notes, discussing what areas worked for you and merit further exploration, and what areas didn't work so you can try to avoid them in the future. It may also be a good idea to check in again a few days to a week after the scene, particularly if this partner is new to you, or if the spanking was unusually physically or emotionally intense.

It's not too rare for one or another partner to notice some "aftershocks" of anger, sadness or guilt after a spanking. It may help simply to know that these feelings are normal, and usually pass within a day or so. Some reassurance from your partner about how terrific the scene was for them can help, too, as can some self-nurturing behavior like a nice hot bath or massage. If these aftershocks seem uncomfortably strong, or persist for more than a couple of days, take a look at the "Troubleshooting" chapter for some help in handling them.

Aftercare helps distinguish the technically competent spankophile from the true artist – and it's fun, too. Don't skimp on it.

10 Troubleshooting

E ven the most skilled and empathetic spankophiles have things go wrong from time to time – freakouts, accidents, unexpected marks, minor injuries, illnesses and more. While many of the precautions I've mentioned in previous chapters will go far in helping to minimize such occurrences, I assure you that problems *will* happen. Here are some strategies for dealing with them when they do.

Emotional Crises
These are probably the single most common mishap that happens in spanking scenes. A bottom may get so deeply into the fantasy that she forgets that this is a consensual scene and gets scared, upset or angry. A spanking may also cause an individual to regress to a deeply childlike, vulnerable state that feels uncomfortable to him, or may even trigger a forgotten memory of trauma or abuse.

The first thing to remember if your partner is having an emotional crisis is that these things happen. Part of the reason we enjoy spanking in the first place is because it lowers some of our emotional barriers and removes some of our armor; sometimes, this process simply goes a bit further than we intended. While it's natural to feel a bit scared and guilty, don't take it too much to heart, unless you were genuinely doing something nonconsensual or non-negotiated.

Next, get to work helping your partner back to a happier frame of mind. Immediately stop spanking him, and release any bondage. If he's wearing any kind of costume or symbols like a collar, find out whether he wants them off or not, and if he does, remove them immediately.

While it can be difficult to conquer your own anxiety and need for reassurance, your main task right now is to be with your partner in a nurturing, non-pushy, non-critical manner. Make sure he's physically warm and comfortable – wrapping him in a cozy blanket can help. Try to get him to eat and drink something (no alcohol, please), since dehydration and low blood sugar can contribute to emotional crises. If he needs to talk, do your best to listen supportively, without getting defensive or guilty. If he needs to cry, hold him if he wants that, or simply stay with him for a while. Stay in physical contact with him if at all possible.

Usually, people begin to recover from an emotional crisis within half an hour or so, and are feeling pretty much better (although, perhaps, still rather raw and vulnerable) within a couple of hours. A crisis that lasts for more than a day or two, or that seems to bring up questions or issues that the individual can't resolve on his own, may indicate that some truly deep and difficult feelings have been stirred up which might require help from a mental health professional to understand and resolve. See the Resource Guide in the back of this book for information about how to find such a professional who will not be judgmental about your partner's interest in spanking.

Physical Injuries

Since it is set up for treatment of minor injuries due to impact and overexertion, sports medicine offers some insights for spanking fans. One good book is listed in the Resource Guide.

Although spanking is far less likely to cause injuries than, say, touch football, people do occasionally get hurt. While this book is not a substitute for professional first aid instruction, here are some methods for dealing with some of the common injuries encountered by spanking folk.

✋ **Welts.** Getting an icebag onto freshly spanked skin can help reduce or eliminate welts. (More about icebags under "Bruises," below.) I have also heard, although I haven't tried it myself, that one or two doses of over-the-counter antihistamine such as diephenhydramine, chlorpheniramine or clemastine can reduce welting. (Read the package carefully; some of these drugs cause drowsiness, or interact badly with other medications.) Welts usually fade within a day or so even if you don't do anything to fix them, although immersion in hot water may cause them to resurface after you think they're gone.

✋ Bruises. If you suspect that unwanted bruises may result from your spanking, place an icebag on the spanked area immediately afterwards. Keep it there until the area starts to go numb, no more than 15 to 20 minutes. Repeat this process every two to four hours for a day or two if possible.

I found out the hard way (during a parade) that exercise during a spanking can increase bruising.

If bruises come up anyway, there is little you can do. Some bottoms swear by an herbal remedy called arnica, which is available in health food stores in both an oral and a rub-on formulation. I have also heard from reliable sources that bruise plasters, available from Asian herbalists, can help bruises heal faster. In a very-worst-case scenario, ultrasound treatments from a sports medicine practitioner will heal bruises quite quickly.

Light or surface bruising is not a problem from a health point of view. If you are deeply or extensively bruised, it's important to drink a lot of water for a couple of days after your scene. The water helps flush the byproducts of broken blood cells out of your system, protecting your kidneys from damage. Some spankees also like to take some extra Vitamin C, Vitamin E and zinc during this period.

Some health practitioners feel that bruising again over an unhealed bruise can damage your body's ability to heal itself.

A bruise that is hard and bulging to the touch is not a medical emergency, but it's not great for your body either.

If the bruise is in a place that you sit directly on, or if it's near your genitals or asshole, I'd have a doctor take a look at it. Be sure to tell your top about it so she knows to take things a little easier next time.

🖐 **Abraded or broken skin.** If clear fluid or blood is leaking from the skin, the skin should be considered broken. (Sometimes even relatively light spankings can break skin, particularly if they strike pimples or other small flaws on the butt.) Broken skin is an opening through which diseases can be transmitted; do not touch anybody else's broken skin without latex or vinyl gloves unless you are absolutely sure that your own skin is unbroken, or the two of you are in a monogamous relationship.

The first thing to do with broken skin is to make sure it doesn't get infected. Clean it twice a day, with an antibacterial soap containing triclosan and with lots of warm water. If the skin is at particularly high risk for infection – if, for example, it is close to the rectum – consider using a topical antibiotic such as Neosporin or Betadine as well. A cream containing lidocaine or benzocaine will help reduce the pain and keep you more comfortable.

For your own comfort as well as for cleanliness, wearing clean, soft cotton underwear for a few days is a good idea; men's boxer shorts are nice in that they don't have elastic that rubs on tender areas. You might also wish to cover the broken skin with gauze and adhesive tape to prevent your clothing from rubbing against it or sticking to it. You will probably figure out on your own that wearing tight or harsh-textured clothing is not such a good idea.

Once the skin is no longer sticky to the touch, keeping it well anointed with a healing moisturizer can decrease itching and promote healing. Some people like aloe vera or Vitamin E oil for this. My personal preference is a

You can buy it in health food stores.

thick moisturizer called Country Comfort, which contains goldenseal, myrrh and other healing herbs.

If skin has been abraded, it will remain more susceptible to abrasion for a long time. I'd steer clear of rough toys or toys with holes for at least a couple of months after your skin has been broken.

🖐 **Cramps.** Being kept in strenuous positions for a long time during a spanking scene can cause muscles to cramp. If someone in your scene develops a muscle cramp, stop immediately and give the person plenty of time to stretch out the cramp. Don't rub it unless they ask you to. Choose a different position when you resume the spanking.

opposite: *the between-the-legs position.*

🖐 **Fainting and seizures.** A spanking can be a physically and emotionally stressful experience. Occasionally, a bottom is overwhelmed by the experience, and faints or has a seizure. You can help prevent this problem by making sure your bottom has had enough to eat before the scene, and by giving her water to drink during the scene. (One of those plastic sports bottles with a straw or valve in the top comes in handy for this.) If your bottom complains of dizziness or nausea, stop the scene immediately and encourage her to lie down with her feet up.

But if she faints anyway, check her heartbeat and breathing; if they're OK, she will almost certainly come to within a minute or two. (A faint that lasts longer than five minutes or so merits a call for an ambulance.) I wouldn't try to go on with a spanking scene after someone has fainted; instead, make her comfortable, give her something to eat and drink once she's able to sit up on her own, and decompress together for a while.

If your partner becomes unresponsive, rigid, and begins to jerk or twitch uncontrollably, that's probably a seizure.

Treatment for seizures (convulsions) is essentially the same. Clear any furniture or breakables out of the way so that your partner doesn't hurt herself, and wait. A seizure that lasts longer than a minute or two, a second

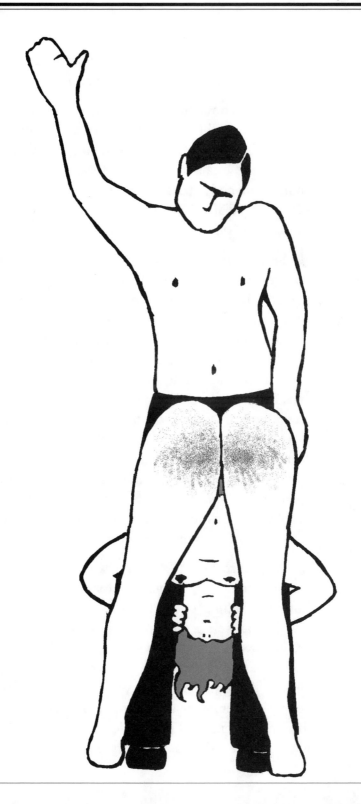

seizure, or a seizure by anyone who's never had one before call for a trip to the emergency room.

✋ **Heat exhaustion.** Both tops and bottoms are susceptible to this problem if they're playing enthusiastically in a warm room. The symptoms to watch out for are dizziness, nausea, rapid heartbeat, and cool clammy skin. If anybody starts to feel these symptoms, stop the scene immediately and give the person plenty of water to drink and perhaps a cool shower.

✋ **Serious injuries.** Any of the following symptoms may represent a serious injury, and call for a trip to the doctor: deep, sharp, or persistent pain in the tailbone; dark urine, bloody urine, or difficulty or pain upon urination; numbness or tingling in any limb that lasts more than an hour or two. See the Resource Guide for help in finding a physician who will treat the injury without being appalled by your spanking interest. It's a good idea to establish a relationship with this doctor *before* you need her.

Health Concerns

If you have any of these problems, a spanking-friendly doctor can also be useful in helping you decide which activities to engage in and which ones to avoid.

While few people are so unhealthy that they shouldn't spank or be spanked at all, some pre-existing health problems do call for adjustments to spanking play. Here are some of the commoner ones:

✋ **Heart trouble.** A bottom with a history of heart trouble should not be placed in stressful positions that impair breathing or circulation. I'd avoid head-down positions as well as standing positions in which the hands are tied overhead. If anybody in the scene complains of dizziness or a pounding heart, stop whatever activity is causing that problem right away. (Since many spanking people also enjoy anal play, it's worth mentioning here that enemas and anal penetration can also be a bit risky with a partner who has a history of heart trouble.)

🖐 **Breathing problems.** A bottom who has asthma, emphysema or other breathing difficulty should not be placed in positions that further impair breathing. Over-the-knee and strongly bent-over positions are particularly likely to cause trouble.

🖐 **Diabetes.** Since diabetes can impair wound healing, it's best not to cause wounds in the first place. Avoid bruising or breaking skin on a bottom with diabetes. Unless she knows for sure that she can handle heavier toys, I'd stick with handspanking, and perhaps a fairly mild leather paddle, on a bottom who has diabetes.

🖐 **Joint problems.** The bottom probably knows better than you what kinds of positions or impact might harm his joints. Follow his directions in choosing what activities to engage in.

It's important to mention here that most spanking aficionadoes spend many years happily spanking or being spanked without encountering a single major problem – I don't want to make it sound as though every spanking is a feat of daredevil risk-taking. Being prepared for trouble is simply a way of helping top and bottom alike to relax and enjoy themselves.

11 Tips, Tricks and Fun Things to Try

Getting bored with the same old whackety-whack? Here are some ideas to spice up or fine-tune your spanking play.

✋ *Get wet.* Many bottoms find that a spanking over wet skin feels much more intense than the same spanking dry. Try giving your partner a nice hot bubble bath, then hauling him out and spanking him while his butt is still all pink and moist. Or use a spray bottle of warm water to keep his backside glistening wet while you spank him.

✋ *Hot creams and liniments.* The feeling of a spanking can be intensified and prolonged by using a mentholatum or capsicum based liniment on the butt before spanking. (A liniment called Heet has a particular cult following.) Some people are allergic to the chemicals in these substances, so it's a good idea to do a patch test on the thin skin of the inner arm 24 hours before your scene. If there is any redness, rash or itching, don't use that liniment on this bottom.

Keep the chemical away from the asshole, genitals, and the crevices between the genitals and thighs – it's not dangerous, but liniments in these tender areas burn too intensely for many bottoms. Similarly, do not use these substances on broken or abraded skin. If the chemical is too intense, immediately apply a lot of anything oily – cold cream, Vaseline, even vegetable oil from the kitchen – and send the bottom off to the shower to shampoo it off (shampoo does a better job of cutting oil than soap does).

If you and your bottom enjoy this sensation, you might experiment cautiously with using a tiny bit of liniment on the outside of her asshole as an incentive to prevent clenching of the cheeks during spanking. (When I say "tiny bit," I mean a dab about half the size of a small pea.)

♨ *Nettles.* Urtification – using stinging nettles to redden, burn and sensitize skin – is a time-honored staple of Victorian spanking porn. If you live in an area where nettles are available, and if your bottom can handle a sensation this intense, it's worth a try. The cautions for nettle play are similar to those for liniment play: patch test first, and keep nettles away from genitals and assholes. I'd start slowly, perhaps using nettles cautiously on a patch a couple of inches square on the bottom's butt and spanking over that, to see how well the bottom can handle the sensation. The sensation should go on burning for a couple of hours, and may feel sort of odd and tingly for a day or two. If that works out well, try a bit more in future sessions.

♨ *"Hey, Keep It Down In There!"* Many spanking fans have to keep the sounds of their play quiet in order to avoid rousing kids or neighbors. There are two parts to this task: one is to keep the noise of the spanks down, the other is to keep the noise of the bottom down.

Broad, flat toys like paddles make a *lot* of noise – a hard paddle stroke can be loud enough to hurt the ears of bystanders. If noise is a concern for you, I'd steer clear of paddles. Somewhere in the middle, noise-wise, are hands and straps. Canes and floggers are relatively quiet, and may be your best bet if you're dealing with paper walls.

As far as keeping your bottom quiet, some bottoms simply don't make much noise: one of the heaviest spanking masochists I know never makes a peep (she has told me that she learned to keep quiet during the years when her own children were young). If your partner is more demonstrative than that, yells, cries and shrieks can be held down by giving him a pillow to hold over his face or something firm but yielding to bite down on (a scrap of heavy leather works well for this). If you want to play with an actual gag, choose something that cannot possibly come loose and work its way into the bottom's throat, and that is small and/or absorbent enough to enable him to swallow his saliva. My personal choice is a large square scarf, folded diagonally into a wide strip, with a large firm knot tied in the middle and the ends tied behind the bottom's head. (And don't forget to agree on a non-verbal safeword –popular ones include humming a bar of a simple tune, knocking three times on a nearby surface, or dropping a held object.)

Mixing spanking with other sensations. A good spanking "wakes up" the skin of the butt, so that other sensations are felt in a sharply focused, highly sensual way. Try delivering a volley of spanks, then caressing the butt with a scrap of fur... or running your fingernails lightly back and forth across the reddened surface... or teasing it with the bristles of your handy hairbrush. Some folks enjoy dripping wax from a plain white paraffin candle (no colored, scented or beeswax candles, please; they burn much too hot for most folks) over already heated skin.

One sensation deserves special mention here: ice. Trailing an ice cube across hot reddened buttflesh is guaranteed to get a gasp from your bottom. You can spank for a while, then use ice to wet down the butt (see "Get Wet" above), then spank some more. Whee!

Games People Play. Many spanking fans enjoy adapting their favorite card or board game to determine who gets spanked, with how many strokes, with which instrument, and so on.

♨ *Plug 'em up.* Inserting a butt plug into your partner's asshole before or during a spanking can greatly increase her sexual stimulation (this trick works on both male and female spankees). Anything inserted into an asshole should have a large flange at its base to keep it from getting pushed too far inside. If she's not used to being anally penetrated, use a very small plug; putting it in a condom (you can tie the condom closed around a small plug, or roll it all the way beyond the flange on a larger one) will make clean-up easier. It's also a good idea to put a towel under your bottom's hips during any kind of anal play, and to keep a couple of small towels or diaper wipes handy for clean-up.

Start by inserting one latex- or vinyl-gloved finger, very well-lubricated with a good water-based lubricant, gradually into her asshole. You'll feel two rings of muscle, which are the outer sphincter and the inner sphincter. Don't force anything; wait until you feel the sphincters relax, usually one at a time, and then gradually move your finger in. Experiment gently with pressing in different directions, moving the finger back and forth, and so on, and watch her reactions. When she seems relaxed and comfortable with one finger, withdraw it, re-lube, and insert two fingers – slowly, gradually. This may be enough for her first time. If she seems stressed or tense, stop after the fingers, and try again another day. On the other hand, if she can relax and enjoy two fingers, you can withdraw them and try gently inserting the plug. Although a stretching feeling, and a feeling of having to defecate, are normal and will fade in a few minutes, nothing should ever feel sharply painful – if it does, stop immediately.

Once the plug is in and she has relaxed again, you can resume the spanking. Try giving a couple of light taps on the base of the plug and see how she reacts to that. Keep an eye on the plug to make sure she isn't pushing it out; if it seems to be trying to sneak away, push it gently back in. Spank away and see how the sensation of anal fullness can contribute to your bottom's enjoyment!

♨ *Masturbation during spanking.* Many women, and quite a few men, can greatly enjoy being allowed – or directed – to masturbate while being spanked. Bottoms of any gender can masturbate in a standing position while you spank their butts. Many women can also masturbate face-down, perhaps with a couple of pillows under their chest and butt, while you spank them. Orgasms achieved in this way tend to be *extremely* intense, so don't expect your bottom to be terribly coherent for a few minutes afterwards.

For a real brain-buster, try handing her (or him, if he enjoys it) a vibrator to use during the spanking. This is intense enough that it's probably best to make sure the bottom is on a bed or soft surface where she won't be hurt if she falls.

On the other hand, some bottoms find that the sensation of the spanking keeps them from reaching orgasm, and/or that the sexual stimulation keeps them from focusing on the spanking. Individual patterns vary; don't push this if it doesn't seem to be working.

♨ *Spanking during intercourse.* While most vaginal and anal intercourse positions don't adapt themselves very well to spanking, there are exceptions. The partner on the bottom during face-to-face fucking may be able to reach up to spank his partner's butt, and the active partner during doggy-style intercourse may enjoy thrusting a couple of times, pulling out for some smacks, and then thrusting again. One excellent position for spanking is for the active partner to lie on his back, with the receptive partner kneeling or lying on top, facing his feet. Although the sweet spot may be hard to reach in this position, most of the rest of the butt is quite marvelously accessible.

♨ *The Crying Game.* Many spanking fantasies end with the "victim" in tears. Yet in the real world, quite a few spankees find it very difficult to cry during a scene (much as they would like to).

I don't have any surefire ways to make a bottom cry. But more than a few bottoms report that they can push themselves to tears by running mental "tapes" of self-pity and victimization – "Poor me... doesn't she know how much this hurts?... How can she do this to me?!" It may help, too, to wait a minute or two longer than usual before using your safeword – some people have a tendency to safeword at exactly the point when they feel their emotions welling up to overwhelm them, so if you hold off for a moment, the next thing you feel might be the need to cry. (Do not, however, delay safewording if you feel that your physical or emotional well-being is genuinely at risk.)

Tops can sometimes help by watching their bottoms for signs of imminent tears, then giving permission for the tears to appear: "That's right, baby, if you need to cry, you go right ahead."

Some bottoms report that they're likelier to cry if a scene includes anal penetration (see "Plug 'Em Up," above) or bondage (see Appendix C). Both of these are worth a try if tears are important to you.

♨ *Invite a friend.* Spanking friends with team spirit may enjoy inviting third, fourth, and even more parties to join their spanking scenes. It's a challenge to the imagination to figure out ways to involve all concerned. Here are a few multi-partner scenes I've seen and participated in:

-   Two spankees stand face-to-face and hold one another, while one or more spankers beat their butts.
-   "Of human bondage" – the spankee is bent over a table or chair while one top holds her hands or arms

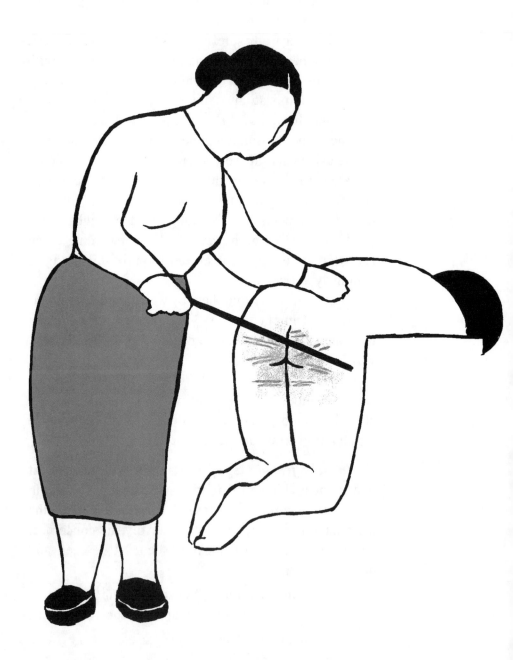

and the other administers the spanking. The two tops may want to change places from time to time.

- A right-handed top can team up with a left-handed top (or a top with a good backhand) and each take one cheek. This scene sometimes resembles a fast-moving game of ping-pong.

- One partner can provide conventional sexual stimulation such as masturbation, oral sex or intercourse to the bottom, while the other spanks him.

These are just a few ideas; the imagination, fantasies and desires of the parties involved will undoubtedly provide more. Have fun!

left: *canes leave a distinctive two-tracked mark...*

12 Conclusion

F or a spanking fan, the end should be the best part, right? So let me just sum up this book by saying that consensual erotic spanking is not violence, not abuse, not a way to degrade or diminish anyone involved. Instead, it is, at its best, a pathway to intimacy and communication, to sharing some of our tenderest, scariest, most vulnerable parts. It's catharsis, nurturance, caring – sometimes even a source of spiritual insight and growth.

By playing with our darkest attractions to power and cruelty, by bringing them out into the light and making them manageable and safe, we gain wholeness and integrity – the chance to accept ourselves and one another as we truly are.

It's time to stop being ashamed. Untold tens of thousands of people share the desire to redden each other's backsides in a loving and consensual manner, and have enhanced their lives and their sexuality by doing so. Why on earth should anybody be ashamed of having more ways to get aroused than their neighbor has? Seems to me that such a person should feel lucky, not guilty.

Everything I've written in this book is simply technique: ways to understand our impulses and to make their passage into reality safer and easier. But the true spirit of erotic spanking can't be written in a book – it comes from the hearts, minds, genitals and butts of those who share this very special, very wonderful desire.

If you are fortunate enough to be such a person, congratulations – and welcome.

Lady Green
December 1996

Finding Others

*O*ne of the biggest challenges facing the would-be spanker or spankee is finding like-minded people – for actual play, or simply for support, friendship and information exchange.

If you're already partnered, do not make the mistake of assuming that your partner will be shocked, frightened or disgusted with your desires: more people share your interest than you might think. On the other hand, there *are* risks involved in telling your partner about your spanking interest – and once you tell, you can't take it back. Still, if you never ask, you'll never find out.

One thing I can tell you for sure is that the subtle-hint route – leaving a hairbrush on the nightstand and then picking a fight, or other such silliness – doesn't work. I've never heard of a single couple discovering a mutually satisfying interest in spanking via this routine.

No, you're going to have to bite the bullet and say the words. If you're interested in topping, you might try saying something like, "You know, it would really turn me on if you'd let me try spanking your bottom lightly sometime." If your urges run more in the bottom direction, try something along the lines of "You know, I've been having some fantasies about being spanked. Could you try smacking my butt lightly sometime during sex and see how that feels?" The idea is to be as non-pushy and non-intimidating as possible, giving your partner the chance to start slowly and see how it feels, and to work your way up gradually with plenty of attention to both partners' comfort. (This gradual approach is for your benefit as well as your partner's – I've heard a lot of stories about well-meaning partners who spanked their spankophile spouses well beyond their limits, thinking that this was what they "really" wanted.) It's a good idea to establish safewords from the very beginning – novice spankers and spankees find it very comforting to know that either partner has a way to communicate immediately if anything goes seriously wrong.

Of course, you may discover that your partner wants absolutely nothing to do with even the lightest spanking games.

This is a difficult problem. You may decide that your spanking desires are best kept as a fantasy. You and your partner may be able to work out some sort of arrangement in which you do your spanking play with someone else, while preserving the primary nature of your relationship. You may decide to spank or be spanked on the sly (which I don't encourage – I've been there and it's awful). Or you may decide that your spanking needs are so strong that you can't stay in a relationship where they can't be met. I encourage you to think any of these steps over *very* carefully, possibly with the help of a nonjudgmental mental health professional, before you do anything you'll regret later.

On a happier note, say you're not already coupled, and that you're looking for a new partner with whom to explore spanking. One possibility is to meet someone in a "vanilla" environment, and try to get them interested in spanking. This can work pretty well – a lot of people have unexplored fantasies in this area – if you are sensitive to their needs and willing to walk away from a relationship that doesn't offer what you're looking for.

If you're like me, an uninhibited extrovert, anybody who's talked to you for more than five minutes knows all about your fantasies, interests and experiences. (If they're still standing there, you've got a hot prospect on your hands.) But most people prefer to introduce the subject of spanking a little later in the acquaintanceship, and a bit more gradually. I think the best time to discuss such matters is at the point when the two of you have established the definite possibility of a romantic interest, but before you have actually had sex. Tentative inquiries, similar to the ones I mentioned above in the section on interesting a current partner, are a good way to start. If your romantic interest isn't totally turned off to the idea, you can negotiate some sort of exploration together. If, however, you're met with disbelief, disgust, ridicule, or a simple firm "thanks but no thanks," cut your losses and begin looking for a more suitable partner.

If you want to restrict your partner-finding to venues where you know that the people you talk to will already have some openness to spanking, your best bet is – duh! – a spanking-oriented environment. The Internet has provided a tremendous number of opportunities for spankophiles to find one another. In Usenet, the soc.subculture.spanking newsgroup is a place for people to post stories, fantasies, queries and experiences. Personal ads belong in alt.personals.spanking. IRC (Internet Relay Chat) provides an environment in which spanking fans can communicate in real-time, and even "play" on-line. Many of the major Internet providers such as America Online and Compuserve also offer spanking-oriented chat rooms and forums. Specialized men-only and women-only spanking groups and mailing lists are available in many of these environments.

Other venues for personal advertising and contact include several of the magazines and newsletters listed in the Resource Guide. Be clear about your interests in terms of gender, intensity, and geographical area.

A few spanking clubs exist around the U.S.; the ones I was able to find out about are listed in the Resource Guide. Several of them put on spanking parties on a regular schedule, often twice a year. Some swing clubs are also open to spanking play, although they might be uncomfortable with very intense spanking. (Many of these environments, sad to say, are not open to heterosexual men without partners, or to gay or bisexual men.)

A tremendous number of general S/M clubs are springing up around the country – men-only, women-only and pansexual. All of them are quite open to spanking play. If you join such a club, you will see many other types of erotic power exchange besides spanking, but nobody will push you to get involved in anything that doesn't interest you. Some spanking fans who attend such clubs find other areas of interest, while others stick strictly to spanking –either is fine, as long as you respect other people's desires as you would want yours respected. I have listed some of the largest and best-known S/M clubs in the Resource Guide.

Remember – just because a potential partner is into spanking doesn't mean they're a good match for you. If someone wants to play in a way that is considerably less intense or more intense than you do, or if they're interested in roles or playstyles that don't work for you, the fact that they enjoy spanking isn't going to matter much. Even more important, a good spanking partner should also be, at minimum, a good friend – someone who shares your values and interests, who you like and enjoy spending time with. Putting up with someone you can't stand simply to get your spanking needs met is a *very* bad idea. Better to fantasize, masturbate and wait for Mr. or Ms. Right.

A final word about finding people to play with. Many men, and more than a few women, get their regular "dose" of spanking from a professional dominant (or, occasionally, a professional submissive). A skilled and empathetic professional can actually be an excellent way to get started with spanking, or to get your needs met while you look for the top or bottom of your dreams. The best professional dominants (most are women, but some are men, often specializing in spanking other men) are extraordinarily good at starting from their client's fantasy and putting their own spin on it, administering spankings tailor-made to the customer's physical and emotional needs. Very few of them provide any form of sexual stimulation for their clients, a precaution which is for your safety as well as theirs.

Finding the right professional usually starts with a search through your local adult paper, or one of the national publications featuring ads from professional dominants and submissives. However, these ads give no clue as to who is a competent and trained professional, and who is a quick-buck artist with no concern for your safety or enjoyment. In seeking a professional dominant or submissive, consider asking the following questions:

Where and by whom were you trained?

What kinds of scenes do you specialize in?

Do you belong to any spanking or S/M clubs?

What kind of equipment, toys and safety gear does your playspace contain?

While it is rude to take up too much of a professional's time on a phone call, any competent professional dominant or submissive should be able to answer these questions clearly and quickly.

If you find a professional who's right for you, treat her with the same courtesy and respect that you would your doctor, dentist, attorney or any other professional. I have heard of professional/client spanking relationships that lasted for years and contained a tremendous amount of mutual affection and respect: to get the intimacy and empathy you want from your spanking play, it's in your best interest to develop this kind of rapport.

Appendix

B

Cleaning Spanking Implements

*A*ny spanking implement that has come into contact with blood, plasma (the clear fluid that oozes from abraded skin), semen, feces or vaginal fluids should be well cleaned before it is used on another bottom. If you're not absolutely positive that a toy hasn't come into contact with these fluids, assume that it has, and clean it.

One solution to this problem is to keep each toy for use on one bottom only. Many bottoms like to own their own toys for use on their own butts.

But if your toys are shared by more than one bottom, you should know how to clean them. Here are some guidelines for keeping your toys clean.

❦ Toys of metal, or manmade materials such as silicon, rubber and many plastics, are a cinch. Just toss them in a solution of nine parts cool water to one part chlorine bleach for half an hour, then rinse them well with running water and dry them. Or, if the toy is heatproof, run it through a regular cycle in the top rack of the dishwasher. If a toy is too large or long for either of these options, wash it with a nonoxynol-9-based toy cleanser such as ForPlay, then rinse and dry it well.

❦ The procedure for cleaning a toy of plant material such as wood or rattan depends on whether or not it is varnished. If it is, you can wash it well with nonoxynol-9-based toy cleanser, rinse it and dry it. (Note: nonoxynol-9 removes some kinds of varnish. If this happens to your toy, sand it smooth with light-grade sandpaper, then revarnish it with a couple of coats of varnish – urethane for inflexible toys like paddles, marine spar varnish for flexible toys like canes.)

Unvarnished toys are difficult to clean. If an unvarnished toy of mine got contaminated with someone's fluids, I'd probably give the bottom that toy for her exclusive use. But if you're determined to hang onto the toy, leaving it in direct sunlight for a couple of days, turning it over to make sure the sunlight reaches all of its surfaces, should kill most of the bugs on it. Or you can sand it very well, starting with heavy sandpaper and moving toward lighter paper until its surface is smooth.

Birches and switches should never be used on more than one bottom – they're too likely to break skin, and they're impossible to clean.

✋ Cleaning leather toys is a bit of a project, but it's not complicated. First, wash the toy well with saddle soap and warm water. Then wipe a thick coat of providone-iodine disinfectant (such as Betadine) all over the surface of the leather. (This disinfectant will stain light-colored leather. I'd keep light-colored leather toys for use in situations where they're not likely to come into contact with body fluids.) Let the toy dry thoroughly, then wipe it clean with a damp cloth, and recondition it with a good-quality hide rejuvenator.

Appendix

C

Combining Bondage With Spanking

Some spanking fans are very turned off by the idea of bondage, while others can't begin to enjoy a spanking until they (or their "victims") are well fastened down.

If you like the idea of adding bondage to your spanking play, I strongly recommend that you buy one or two of the basic S/M texts listed in the Resource Guide, or attend classes or workshops put on by your local S/M club. Improperly done bondage can be dangerous in and of itself, and bondage also increases the risks of other kinds of problems that might take place during your scene.

At a minimum, if you want to experiment with bondage, please keep in mind the following guidelines:

❦ Use materials that are broad enough not to cut into skin or muscle. (Nylon stockings, often the first choice of novices, are notorious for causing problems.) If you're using rope, use soft, relatively thick rope, and place several coils around each limb. Better yet, invest in a good set of leather or nylon restraints (*not* metal handcuffs).

❦ Never tie anybody up unless you know exactly how you'd get them loose in case of an emergency such as a fire, panic attack or sudden illness. Don't assume that you can untie a knot quickly under emergency conditions – knots jam. Keep a knife or scissors, strong and sharp enough to cut quickly through your bondage materials, within arm's reach; paramedic shears, available in medical supply stores, are ideal. If you have someone standing with his hands tied overhead, think about how you'd get that person down if he suddenly fainted. (Hint: riding supply and marine supply stores sell an item called a "panic snap" that can be released under pressure.)

❦ Do not place restraints tightly over places where nerves or blood vessels are close to the surface of the skin. The insides and sides of wrists and the backs of knees are particularly vulnerable. And I hope I don't have to tell you not to place any bondage material across the front of anyone's neck.

♨ Be aware that emergencies happen: bottoms have emotional flashbacks or physical illnesses; fires, earthquakes and hurricanes don't always respect your desire for a nice happy spanking; children and family members sometimes need immediate attention. A top who places a bottom in bondage is taking responsibility for his welfare in these and other emergency situations. Equip your play space with emergency lighting, fire extinguishers and a first-aid kit. I also strongly encourage tops (and, for that matter, bottoms) to obtain training in basic first aid and cardiopulmonary resuscitation; your bottom's emotional and physical well-being is in your hands.

Appendix

D

Resource Guide

In Case of Problems

For a list of physicans, chiropractors, therapists and other professionals who will not be judgmental about your spanking interest, visit the Kink-Aware Professionals website at
www.bannon.com/kap

If you are being spanked against your will and want help in preventing it, or if you are spanking someone against their will and want help in stopping:
National Domestic Violence Hotline
(800) 799-SAFE
or check the front of your phone book for local resources

For help with care of minor spanking-related injuries, this is a good reference book:
Sports Medicine for Coaches & Trainers
Edward J. Shahady, M.D., & Michael J. Petrizzi, M.D.
University of North Carolina Press, Chapel Hill, NC

If you have general questions about spanking or other forms of erotic behavior:
San Francisco Sex Information
(415) 989-7374

Spanking Clubs

This is far from an exhaustive list of the spanking clubs throughout the U.S. Many are small, local, and do not widely publicize their activities. Your local S/M club or alternative newspaper may be able to put you in touch with a club near you... or try entering the search terms "spanking," "club" and the name of your city into your favorite seasrch engine. Please note that most clubs which accept both men and women tend to be rather conservative about admitting single men; you'll do better if you can find a female partner to accompany you.

Crimson Moon
"Men who wish to play with other men will not find our group to their liking." Parties every other month. Formerly TSOSF.
Box 95484
Palatine, IL 60095-0484
http:/www.crimson-moon-ltd.com

Northeast Erotic Spanking Society (NESS)
enclose a stamped self-addressed envelope and $3 for newsletter and application form
NESS/TEP
P.O. Box 540441
Waltham MA 02454-0441

Shadow Lane
Semi-annual spanking conferences for women and couples, usually held in Southern California.
(818) 985-9151
http://www.shadowlane.com

General S/M Clubs

Again, this is a list which is far from complete – hundres of S/M clubs have sprung up across the U.S. and worldwide. These, however, are some of the largest, and may be able to put you in touch with a club nearer you, or with a male-only or female-only club if that is your preference. Please remember that while S/M may include many activities besides spanking, many S/M folks are also avid spanking fans.

National Leather Association
Pansexual but membership is primarily gay & lesbian. Chapters in many cities.
4031 Wycliff Ave #958
Dallas, TX 75219
www.nla-i.com

The Eulenspiegel Society
The oldest pansexual S/M club in the U.S. In addition to its regular programs, it also maintains a Spanking special interest group.
P.O. Box 2783
New York, NY 10003
(212) 388-7022
www.tes.org

The Society of Janus
P.O. Box 411523
San Francisco, CA 94141-1523
(415) 292-3222
http://www.soj.org

Black Rose
(Washington DC area)
www.br.org

Books

Nonfiction

This is, as far as I know, the only nonfiction how-to book entirely about spanking. However, several of the more general S/M books out there contain excellent spanking material. Greenery Press publishes several of the best (if I do say so myself); check the back page of this book for our listings. In addition, these books are recommended:

Consensual Sadomasochism: How to Talk About It and How to Do It Safely
William A. Henkin, Ph.D., and Sybil Holiday, CCSSE
Daedalus Press, San Francisco

Different Loving: An Exploration of the World of Sexual Dominance and Submission
Brame, Brame & Jacobs
Villard Books, NY

A Guide to the Correction of Young Gentlemen
I include this here with some hesitation – I think it has more to do with fiction than with how-to. Still, a lot of the ideas are exciting. I suggest you use it as a source of arousal rather than information.
Delectus Books, London

Learning The Ropes
Race Bannon
Daedalus Press, Los Angeles

Leathersex
Joseph Bean
Daedalus Press, Los Angeles

Screw the Roses, Send Me the Thorns
Philip Miller & Molly Devon
Mystic Rose Books, Fairfield, CT

Sensuous Magic: A Guide for Adventurous Couples
Pat Califia
Cleis Press, San Francisco

Fiction

There are about three zillion hot erotic novels that are either entirely or mostly about spanking, and I wouldn't dream of trying to list even a fraction of them here. Most of the current stuff is being published either by Masquerade Books (or its imprints, Rhinoceros, Rosebud and a few more), or by Blue Moon; a visit to a good bookstore or erotic boutique should net you a handful at least. I do want to mention a couple of erotic spanking novels that have become classics and have been widely enjoyed by many spanking fans.

The Art of Spanking (graphic novel)
Enard, illustrated by Milo Manara
NBM Press, NY

The Beauty Trilogy (The Claiming of Sleeping Beauty, Beauty's Punishment, Beauty's Release)
Anne Rice writing as A.N. Roquelaure
Dutton Books, NY

Harriet Marwood, Governess
Anonymous
Masquerade Books, NY

My Private Life: Real Experiences of a Dominant Woman
This is actually a memoir, not a novel. Real-world experiences of a respected Southern California spanker and dominant.
Daedalus Press, Los Angeles

Spanking in the Mainstream Media

*There are so many **mainstream movies** which include spanking that a complete list would almost be a book of its own. However, some favorites of spanking fans include John Wayne and Maureen O'Hara's "McClintock!" and James Garner's "Tank." Watch for robot spanking in "Class of 2000," public school caning in*

"If..." and "Flirting," and a deeply bizarre spanking scene with Christopher Lloyd and Sandra Bernhard (!) in "Track 29."

Romance novels *that contain some spanking scenes include Heather Graham's "Love Not a Rebel," Catherine Creel's "Texas Torment," "Captive Flame" and "Texas Spitfire," Lane Harris's "Devil's Love," Judith McNaught's "Whitney, My Love," and several novels by Karen Robards. (Thanks to the online folks who provided this information.)*

Science fiction and fantasy novels *that have spanking scenes include almost everything by Sharon Green or John Norman, many novels by Robert Heinlein, and Johanna Lindsey's "Warrior Woman." Also, watch especially for John Varley's novella "The Persistence of Vision," which contains one of the most moving spanking scenes ever written.*

Magazines

Primarily Spanking
CF Publications (also offers novels)
www.cfpub.com

Red Tails (gay male; also offers videos)
www.manshandfilms.com

Stand Corrected
Shadow Lane Productions (also offers videos)
http://www.shadowlane.com

General BDSM

Prometheus
The quarterly publication of The Eulenspiegel Society.
P.O. Box 2783
New York, NY   10003
(212) 388-7022
www.tes.org

Electronic Resources

The Internet newsgroups soc.sexuality.spanking and alt.sex.spanking.moderated are reliable sources of information and connection, with a far-above-average number of well-written and literate stories and poems on the subject of spanking.

Personal ads should not appear here, but are welcome on alt.personals.spanking.

Many of the large Internet providers such as America OnLine, Compuserve and The Microsoft Network also provide special chat rooms and forums for spanking fans. Try doing a keyword search on the word "spank" and see what comes up.

For national personal ads, consider www.spanking.com, a website exclusively for spanking ads. You could also take a look at www.adultfriendfinders.com and www.adult.com, both specializing in kinky and alternative sex.

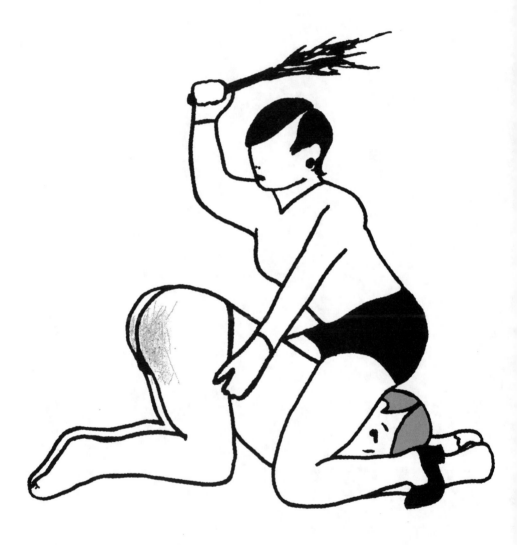

Opposite: *The bottom is in the knee-to-chest position while the top straddles his shoulders with a birch. Notice that he is wearing a leather g-string,which will help protect his testicles.*

Other Books from Greenery Press

GENERAL SEXUALITY

Big Big Love: A Sourcebook on Sex for People of Size & Those Who Love Them
Hanne Blank $15.95

The Bride Wore Black Leather... And He Looked Fabulous!: An Etiquette Guide for the Rest of Us
Andrew Campbell $11.95

The Ethical Slut: A Guide to Infinite Sexual Possibilities
D. Easton & C.A. Liszt $16.95

A Hand in the Bush: The Fine Art of Vaginal Fisting
Deborah Addington $13.95

Health Care Without Shame: A Handbook for the Sexually Diverse & Their Caregivers
Charles Moser, Ph.D., M.D. $11.95

The Lazy Crossdresser
Charles Anders $13.95

Look Into My Eyes: How to Use Hypnosis to Bring Out the Best in Your Sex Life
Peter Masters $16.95

Supermarket Tricks: More than 125 Ways to Improvise Good Sex
Jay Wiseman $11.95

Turning Pro: A Guide to Sex Work for the Ambitious and the Intrigued
Magdalene Meretrix $16.95

When Someone You Love Is Kinky
D. Easton & C.A. Liszt $15.95

BDSM/KINK

The Bullwhip Book
Andrew Conway $11.95

A Charm School for Sissy Maids
Mistress Lorelei $11.95

Family Jewels: A Guide to Male Genital Play and Torment
Hardy Haberman $12.95

Flogging
Joseph W. Bean $11.95

Jay Wiseman's Erotic Bondage Handbook
Jay Wiseman $16.95

The Loving Dominant
John Warren $16.95

Miss Abernathy's Concise Slave Training Manual
Christina Abernathy $11.95

The Mistress Manual: The Good Girl's Guide to Female Dominance
Mistress Lorelei $16.95

The New Bottoming Book
D. Easton & J.W. Hardy $14.95

Sex DIsasters... And How to Survive Them
Charles Moser, Ph.D., M.D., and Janet W. Hardy $16.95

The Sexually Dominant Woman: A Workbook for Nervous Beginners
Lady Green $11.95

The Topping Book: Or, Getting Good At Being Bad
D. Easton & C. A. Liszt $11.95

FICTION FROM GRASS STAIN PRESS

The 43rd Mistress: A Sensual Odyssey
Grant Antrews $11.95

Haughty Spirit
Sharon Green $11.95

Love, Sal: letters from a boy in The City
Sal Iacopelli, ill. Phil Foglio $13.95

Murder At Roissy
John Warren $11.95

The Warrior Within (part 1 of the Terrilian series)
Sharon Green $11.95

The Warrior Enchained (part 2 of the Terrilian series)
Sharon Green $11.95

Please include $3 for first book and $1 for each additional book to cover shipping and handling costs, plus $10 for overseas orders. VISA/MC accepted. Order from:

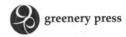 greenery press

1447 Park St., Emeryville, CA 94608
toll-free 888/944-4434   http://www.greenerypress.com